*the other side of the*
# RAINBOW

*Mickey Antu–Urias*

# *the other side of the* RAINBOW

## Memoirs of a
## Brain Aneurysm Survivor

TATE PUBLISHING *& Enterprises*

Published by Tate Publishing & Enterprises, LLC
127 E. Trade Center Terrace | Mustang, Oklahoma 73064 USA
1.888.361.9473 | www.tatepublishing.com

Tate Publishing is committed to excellence in the publishing industry. The company reflects the philosophy established by the founders, based on Psalm 68:11,
*"The Lord gave the word and great was the company of those who published it."*

Book design copyright © 2011 by Tate Publishing, LLC. All rights reserved.
*Cover design by Kristen Verser*
*Interior design by Joel Uber*

Published in the United States of America

ISBN: 978-1-61739-929-9
1. Biography & Autobiography; Medical
2. Biography & Autobiography; Personal Memoirs
11.02.08

*In Loving Memory*

SIFREDO ANTU
MAY 29, 1937 – JULY 8, 2009

# DEDICATION

To the loves of my life,
Joel, Eric, and Kyle,
Because of *you*…I couldn't let go.
Because of *God*…I wasn't let go.

# ACKNOWLEDGMENTS

My wish was to include the many, many professionals, family members, and friends who played roles in both my survival and my ongoing recovery. Since there were indeed so many involved, I apologize in advance if I have omitted anyone. You know who you are, and you are loved and appreciated more than my simple words can express.

God
Dad
Joel, Eric, and Kyle
Frances Antu and Toni Antu-Rocha
*San Antonio Express-News*
H.E.B. Grocery Company

Dr. Arnold B. Vardiman
Dr. Donald Hilton
Dr. John D. Hermann
Dr. Sergio A. Garcia
Dr. Charles P. Andrews
Dr. James H. Wright
Dr. James E. Dix
Dr. Obinna H. Ozigbo
Dr. Vu Nguyen Vu
Dr. Vincent Caldarola
Dr. Randall Bell
Dr. Karl Swann
Dr. Maria Chapa
Dr. Michael Scott Figueroa
Dr. John Green III
Dr. Steven Wegert
Dr. James Gilley
Dr. Michael Lane
Dr. Richard A. Benedikt
Dr. David W. Bynum
Dr. Martin J. Wiesenthal
Dr. John Luther
Dr. Jorge Munoz
Dr. Philip Onghai
Healthsouth RIOSA
Maria T. Byron, RN
Caroline Kalkhoff-McKinney, RN
Audrey J. Wilson, LVN
Emanuel C. Graham, RN
Diana Evetts, RN

Catalina L. Corona, NS
Daren S. Stroud, LVN
Alexandra Orospe, GN
Nancy L. Stephan, RN
Lori K. Wynn, RN
Joseph Millet III, RN
Sharon Watson, RN
Jennie M. Wackler, RN
Tiffany Cooper, RN
Autumn L. Carnesi, RN
Nerrisa Persad, RN
Kenneth R. Drummond, GN
Elizabeth Berg, GN
Brian J. Moczygemba, RN
Gwendolyn Mullinix, RN
Janelle M. Geary, RN
Jessica D. Eden, RN
Kathleen M. Carter, RN
Jessica D. Eden, RN
Diane Williams, RN
Diana McCartney, RN
Oriana C. Gonzalez, RN
Lynn McDowell, RN
Tina L. Barton, RCP
Elva P. Gomez, PCA
Beverly J. Fischer, RCP
Nina Y. Vargas, PCA
Joven Moselina, OTR
Roel Zavala, PTA
Jessica Estrada, PT

Ismael Garibay, Chaplain
Botchke & Handlers
Valerie Martinez, EMT
Dena Spring, EMT
Chris Thomas, EMT
K. B. Hallmark, EMT
Matthew Hayden, EMT

Brain Aneurysm Foundation, Boston, MA
San Antonio Chapter – Brain Aneurysm Support Group
Dr. Christopher J. Koebbe

While it may take a "village to raise a child"...
I'll always appreciate that it takes a passionate,
dedicated "galaxy" of professionals to care for a
brain injury patient.
My Eternal Thanks

# TABLE OF CONTENTS

Introduction                                15

Yesteryear                                  17

A Perfect Day                               21

Without Warning – The Rupture               27

Alive on Arrival                            37

Home Away From Home                         43

Scared Doesn't Begin to Cover It            77

Rebuilding My Faith                         85

Helping Hands                               89

Awareness – What Everyone Should Know      119

My Perfect Rainbow                         129

# INTRODUCTION

*"There are only two ways to live your life.*
*One is as though nothing is a miracle.*
*The other is as though* everything *is a miracle."*
Albert Einstein

God puts the right people, in the right place, at the right time. I was never more convinced of this than the day I could have, would have, and perhaps should have died. Looking back, the events of March 1, 2008, were nothing short of a miracle. Don't call me lucky. Call me blessed. Extremely blessed. Someone once said, "Only fools chase rainbows." Most of my existence has been on *this* side of the rainbow. Only after my near-death experience, and overcoming the fear that would paralyze me for months afterward, would I venture over to *The Other Side of the Rainbow*—you know, that imaginary, fairy-tale place where a pot of gold supposedly awaits you? Until then, there would be tears. Many, many tears.

*And then came the laughter…*

Sadly, this is no fairy tale. It is a very real story of surviving a ruptured brain aneurysm and coming to terms with the question, "why me?"

# YESTERYEAR

*"Life's challenges are not supposed to paralyze you;
they're supposed to help you discover who you are."*
Bernice Johnson Reagon

Why does one ask "why?" Like the proverbial three-year-old, I always have and will always continue to ask "why?" when an explanation is warranted. It is quite possible that we are simply inquisitive creatures. It is also possible that we don't understand or don't agree with whatever we continue to question. In many cases, I am convinced that it is the shear disbelief of some of the events that have transpired in my life.

The older I became, the more in control I needed to be of my destination. As the product of divorced parents by age eight and the oldest of three sisters, my life would take on many colors. Why was my childhood so troubled in spite of my father's endless efforts to make a good life for us?

As a child, I even questioned why I was so accident prone and always getting hurt. Not just scrapes and bruises, although there were an abundance of those as well.

One of the many nightmares parents endure is that of their child getting hurt. My parents held up remarkably well in spite of all of the injuries I sustained in my youth, the worst of which was a bicycle accident that produced a skull fracture. Somebody really should have told me you don't stop a runaway bike by riding it directly into a parked car. Who knew? I was going downhill, having a jolly good time, until the chain came off of this deathtrap. In my own defense, I was only six years old and the reasoning of this six-year-old was that the parked car would make the bike stop. What I had not calculated was flying off upon impact. It was nothing short of a miracle that I didn't crash right through the windshield. Unfortunately, my head made contact with the curb upon landing.

Next was the time my hand got stuck in one of the first electric laundry wringers. Yes, this really can and did happen. Just when you thought these things only happened in cartoons. One of my most vivid of recollections is that of my dad running out the front door of our house in his boxers! Imagine someone waking you from a sound sleep to tell you your first-born has a fence board hanging out of her forehead and is bleeding all over the place. All this fun we experienced before my ninth birthday. Why? Simply put, I was just a clumsy daredevil wannabe with no true "superhero" skills.

As the oldest of three girls, I had no one to emulate and, therefore, had to set my own standards. Apparently, I didn't raise the bar very high for my two younger sisters.

It wasn't only physical pain I questioned, but broken hearts too. Why did bad things happen to good people? At age twelve, I would ask our church pastor why God allowed wars and why people had to die such horrible deaths. Why did some kids not have moms or dads? Again, why, why, why?

By the age of twenty-three, I was married and the mother of the most adorable baby boy one could ever hope for. Unfortunately, this marriage would not endure our foolish youthfulness. When Eric was a mere ten months old, his father and I called it quits. After a brief but failed reconciliation, I would find myself the single mother of a two-year-old toddler and headed to divorce court. Why? Character would begin to take shape, as well as my fight for survival. This would be a no-holds-barred fight for survival. I would not fail my child.

Looking back now, it turns out those were much simpler times after all.

Fast-forward twenty-five years. I need to believe this self-defense mechanism would play a pivotal role in my survival when faced with the uncertainty of life or death.

My faith and my walk with God would solidify this theory.

# A PERFECT DAY

*Attitude to me is more important than facts. It is more important than the past, than education, than money, than circumstances, than failures, than success, than what other people think, say or do. It is more important than appearance, gift or skill. It will make or break a company...a church... a home. The remarkable thing is we have a choice every day regarding the attitude we will embrace for that day...I am convinced that life is 10 percent what happens to me and 90 percent how I react to it. And so it is with you...we are in charge of our attitudes.*

Charles Swindol

It was a beautiful, spring-like Saturday morning, although spring had not officially begun. The kind of day you don't mind jumping out of bed early for, even if it is a rare day off. Besides, I would need to head to my office on Sunday to complete two separate projects with deadlines fast approaching. There were never enough hours in the day. I would relish this single day off for the week. This had become an all too familiar pace, so today would be special. It would be a day filled with relaxation and no worries. What could possibly go wrong on a day filled with such extraordinary beauty?

My hometown of San Antonio is notorious for short, mild winters and long, brutal summers. "Hot" and "hotter-n-hell" are the two seasons we typically experience here in south Texas. Somewhere in between we get about six weeks of picture-perfect weather. Winters are uneventful, and snow is pretty much an urban myth. Many college-age students have never even seen snow in this region, if they were born and raised in the Alamo city.

So my plan was to not waste a minute of this glorious day. Eric, the older of my two sons, had already moved out of our house, and seventeen-year-old Kyle had his own agenda with a part-time job and a very busy social calendar. After the purchase of his '96 Honda Civic, we saw little of him. Home by curfew was all we asked. A decent young man, he not only enjoyed working for his own spending money but turned out to be quite the popular kid as well.

While my husband, Joel, slept in, I would handle a couple of chores. Joel, the love of my life, owned and operated his own mobile deejay business, which kept him out very late and entitled him to sleep late. With a standing Friday night gig at a local sports bar, he usually wasn't home until well after 2:30 a.m. on Saturday. He spent the next couple of hours unloading his truck and unwinding. By the time he was off to bed, it was typically 4:00 a.m. Often times he was coming to bed as I was arising for the day.

Saturday night gigs were also a staple, usually booked solid for the month. This particular Saturday was an exception. Or was it divine intervention? For on this fateful Saturday night, there was no bride and groom, no debutante, and no birthday or corporate event to cater to. We would spend a rare Saturday night together.

Much to my delight, Joel awoke early all on his own. In my mind, I had already outlined our day. A few chores, but seriously, on a day like this, it would really be just a few. We would then head out to our preferred mall, The Forum. This mall was one of the first outdoor malls in the area—chock-full of retailers, eateries, and just about anything else you might need. A favorite pastime, we would walk in and out of the usual twenty-plus retailers we favored. Eventually, we would grab a light snack and wander over to the local Starbucks for a caffeine-boost. There, we would sit at a sidewalk table where I could smoke, and we might people watch. The picture-perfect weather would bring people out in droves. We especially favored watching the little ones who were accompanied to the Baskin Robbins strategically located next to Starbucks. Joel and I got such a kick out of small children, most likely because we were on the verge of becoming empty nesters. We pretty much already were. At seventeen, Kyle would grace us with his presence long enough to eat what wasn't nailed to the floor and sleep. He was definitely a typical teenager; if he wasn't eating or sleeping, he was usually on his way out the door—off to school or work, out skateboarding, or just hanging out with friends.

It didn't appear we would have any grandchildren in the near future, as Eric had already shared with us that he didn't care to have any kids. Just a phase, I told myself. Surely he would change his mind. He is after all, only twenty-five. Lots of couples are waiting until later in life to start families, wanting to complete educations, getting established in careers, and sowing wild oats. Whatever the reason, it has simply become more commonplace to wait. Still, I thought about babies often and daydreamed about if and when we would have grandkids to help care for, cuddle, play with, and so on. Joel interrupted my trance and asked, "Are you ready to head back out?" We still had a few stores to patronize before making our way back home.

Walking back toward the main shopping strip, we encountered a couple of good friends, Liz and Mando. I have a lot of "favorite" people, and Liz and Mando rank high on that list. Liz and I have worked together for many years, and Mando also worked at the paper before moving on to greener pastures. This chance encounter remains with me still.

About an hour later, Joel and I would begin to wrap up our day trip, as we both conceded we were getting pretty tired. We decided to have dinner, go home, and watch a movie. It had been a long and satisfying day.

We arrived home around 6:45 p.m. Kyle was still at work, bussing tables at the Texas Roadhouse, the same restaurant where his older brother, Eric, was a server. Toby, our four-year-old Beagle mix, was both happy to see us and annoyed that we had been gone so long. He gave us a dirty-dog look and made himself comfortable on his bed, which just so happened to double as our sofa.

We prepared to settle in for a quiet evening. When Joel began his deejay business, we knew there would be sacrifices to be made. It was still a challenge because we've always enjoyed each other's company so much. Perhaps it was because our work schedules are as opposite as day and night. As a matter of fact, they are day and night. I work days and sleep at night; he works nights and sleeps during the day. Absence really does make the heart grow fonder.

Once we arrived home, Joel was off to the master bath to change into his pajama bottoms, and I found my favorite nightshirt to wear. We met back in the living room, much to the delight of Toby.

*Maria, la del Barrio*, a Mexican novella (soap opera) we had been watching on DVD, was prepped for viewing. This was a nineties soap we had recorded on VHS and watched early on, before losing track of time and episodes. Now that Joel found the complete season on DVD, commercial-free and with English subtitles, we were ready to get answers to all the questions we had been left with. Before we got comfortable in our his and hers recliners, Joel wanted to test the iPod conversion kit he had purchased earlier in the day. While he was outside in his truck, playing with his new toy, I returned a call to my sister Toni in Illinois.

I stepped outside on our back porch, lit a cigarette, and dialed her number. We usually played phone tag, so I was surprised when she answered her cell phone. With our busy lives, we didn't talk often enough, and traveling to and from posed even more of a challenge. Had it not been for an unfortunate emergency trip she made to Texas, I would not have seen her for a couple of years.

# Without Warning –
# The Rupture

*Do not fear, for I am with you; do not be dismayed,*
*for I am your God. I will strengthen you and help*
*you; I will uphold you with my righteous right hand.*
Isaiah 41:10

Although I have never really considered myself a superstitious person, posted on our refrigerator door was a tiny slip of paper with a fortune from a long-since eaten fortune cookie. Somehow, out of the hundreds of fortune cookies cracked open and read aloud over the years, I must have believed this one in particular to be an epiphany. It read, "The Road Ahead of You is Long…Drive Safely."

My memory of talking on the phone with Toni—or listening, as we all joked, because Toni has always been such a chatterbox—is as clear as a bell. We hadn't been on the phone for more than five minutes when her voice began fading in and out, on and off. It sounded like listening to someone talk while my head was submerged under water. Wasn't quite sure if I was just tired or if she was not positioning her phone properly. You know how when you try to hold a three-inch cell phone on your shoulder so you can talk and multitask loading the dishwasher, the washer or dryer, or attempting to water the plants? The poor connection continued. Maybe it was *my* cell phone. It was, after all, five years old by now. That's like 180 in cell phone years. When able to, I interrupted Toni and told her I would call her back the next day. We ended our conversation as we always did. "Okay, sis, I'll talk to you later. Take care. I love you."

No sooner had my phone been flipped shut, and without any warning, I experienced the worst pain I had ever felt in my life!

"What the hell?" I recall saying out loud, as though the cause of the pain would reveal itself to me. Was I just hit on the side of my head, blunt force, with a baseball bat? Could it have been a claw hammer?

A burning sensation arose in my nose and throat, but it was the pain in my head that alerted immediate panic. Had I been shot in the back of my head? So extreme was this pain, I turned around to see if there was somebody standing behind me. There wasn't of course, but something else was wrong—very, very wrong.

The pain was excruciating. The kind of pain that might cause one to lose consciousness, but I didn't.

Not just then. I knew right away I had to get to Joel. He could help me, but I had to reach him first, and he was still sitting in his truck, parked in the driveway.

Holding on to my head and squeezing it tightly seemed to provide a miniscule bit of relief. It felt as though my head would burst. At the time, I couldn't begin to imagine what was happening. I didn't have a clue. What I did know was this: I had to make it from the backyard, through the house, and finally out the front door to the driveway. Our house isn't large by any stretch of the imagination, but for every step I took forward, it appeared I fell two steps back. By the grace of God, I remained conscious. That was about to change.

I bumped into and tripped over furniture through-out the house for what seemed like an eternity. When I fell down, I would get up. Whatever body part I hit on any given fall would not be felt until days later. Letting go of my head was not an option; the pain was searing. I finally made my way to the front door. All I could focus on was getting to Joel. He would know what to do. As bad as the pain was, it was going to get worse. Much worse. Fear was already consuming me. "Please Lord, help me…" I began to pray out loud. "Help me get help."

Slowly, I reached down, turned the doorknob, and opened the door. The driveway and his fire engine red pickup truck both appeared to be on the other side of the street! An optical illusion brought on by unimagi-nable pain and sheer terror. As I approached the truck,

Joel looked up and instantly recognized something was not right. When he asked, I explained my head was suddenly, and without provocation, hurting worse than anything I had ever felt. Try as I might, to this day, I have not been able to forget that relentless pain. Amazingly, I could speak. Then the screaming began. Blood curdling screaming that would continue until I would lose consciousness.

Joel's knee-jerk reaction was to get me into his truck so he could drive me to the emergency room. In spite of the pain, the fear, and the uncertainty, I knew this was not a practical offer or a reasonable solution. This could be a mistake of massive proportions.

"Call 911," I said as he jumped out of the truck to accompany me back inside the house. The temperature was dropping outside, and I was barefoot with a nightshirt on. Somewhere between the backyard and driveway, I had lost my slippers.

As we made our way back up the sidewalk and into the house, I screamed in agony.

One of our neighbors, who had been sitting out in her backyard, called the Sheriff's Department to report "a woman screaming."

Back inside the house, Joel positioned me at the end of the sofa and immediately dialed 911. The time was 8:37 p.m. Within the course of one solitary hour, my world had been turned upside down and inside out.

While still on the phone, Joel observed me leaning to my left as I began to slide off the slick leather sofa. Unbeknownst to us at the time, I would now begin to display a common symptom of a subarachnoid hemorrhage, that of uncontrollable emesis (vomiting). This was going to present a whole new set of problems, especially because I was slipping in and out of consciousness.

Joel managed to maintain his composure as he continued his communication with 911. While doing so, he now held on to me as I made the inevitable descent from the sofa to our cold, hard, ceramic living-room floor.

The screaming would continue while Joel spoke to the emergency dispatcher. He answered questions for what seemed like an eternity, in slow motion and in reverse. Time tends to stand still when you experience pain, and this was no ordinary pain. Finally the call was completed. He reassured me the dispatcher estimated the first response team would be at our residence in approximately seven minutes. That sounded very promising, I vaguely remember thinking. Although I was aware of being on the floor, I had no memory of having fallen from the sofa. Nor do I have any recollection of vomiting all over the floor and myself.

Where was my faithful four-legged companion, Tobias Urias?

Joel ran out the front door to get help. He bolted across the street to retrieve our neighbor, Chuck. He wanted to get me back on the sofa and was going to enlist Chuck's help. Joel must have already been out of his mind with worry and needed a support system with him while he waited for the medical response unit to arrive. Seconds later, as the two of them were running back across the street, the first of two ambulances arrived. It was 8:47 p.m. Joel, Chuck, and the first set of EMT's raced through the front door, past the foyer and to the living room where I remained on the floor. In hindsight, I can only imagine what must have gone through the minds of everyone who walked into my house, with me lying on the floor, covered in vomit. Did she overdose on drugs? Could she have food poisoning? There were certainly no visible signs of trauma. No blood to be *seen*. The emergency workers placed me directly on the gurney so they could begin their assessments.

One of the final images I recall, from what should have been the very comfort of my own home, is that of several people standing over me. Chuck's wife, Pat, and daughter, Chelsea, had now rushed over. The crew from the second ambulance had come into the house and waited for instructions. I would continue to slip in and out of consciousness.

Once strapped to the gurney, the short distance from my living room to the ambulance would prove to be a long and very uncomfortable transport. Just when I thought there was no pain greater than what I already felt, the wheels on the gurney would encounter every groove between the tiles on our floor, every crack in the sidewalk, and finally the descent from the curb to the street. Things one would probably not take notice of on an ordinary day. This was a far-from-ordinary experience. Without doubt, I would have felt that gurney roll over a blade of grass.

The pain cannot truly be described. The instant onset of pain brought on by a rupture is referred to as a "Thunderclap." A better comparison would be hard to come by.

Dr. Christopher Koebbe, a neurosurgeon acquaintance and the medical consultant to our support group, would later shed some light with this analogy: "The pain/damage of a brain bleed is comparable to hitting your head on the windshield of a vehicle that has slammed into a cement barrier, traveling at eighty miles per hour, without any external signs of trauma suffered by the brain!"

The medics moved fast. If their suspicions were correct, there was little time to spare. The gurney was loaded into the ambulance and, with one final jolt, locked into place. I was very frightened, extremely cold, most certainly in shock, and already worried about Joel and the boys. *What on earth is wrong with me?* Shivering to the point of convulsing, the last audible sentence I heard from one of the paramedics was "I'm going to start a line on you, sweetie. You're going to be okay, and everything is going to be fine." As convincing as this sounded coming from an extremely calm medic, the pain in my head told another story. Once again, the vomiting began. This time I do remember. It was uncontrollable, projectile vomit. This was not "sick-to-your-stomach" vomiting. I never felt it coming on, and there was no will to control it or fight it off. Suction wands were in and out of my mouth in a fury. The EMTs from the second ambulance were also in the back of this "bus" I had been loaded on to. They all worked in unison, as the risk of drowning in my own vomit had become another concern that needed their immediate attention and intervention.

Remember, God puts the right people, in the right place, at the right time. Another expression I've heard for most of my life is "God doesn't give you any more than you can handle."

True to this expression, I lost consciousness again. Before the ambulance ever pulled away from the front of our home, I was in for the fight of my life. I would also lose the ability to remember most of the events of the next ninety-six hours, and only sporadically recall the next three weeks spent in the hospital.

Our subdivision is located between San Antonio and Converse, Texas, a small suburb—population 17,500. Our house is approximately seventeen doors down from the Converse zip code, and in these parts, we are considered "county." Once 911 had been dispatched, I had an ambulance from each of these jurisdictions at my disposal—one from Bexar County, and the other courtesy of the City of Converse. Did you ever take someone or something for granted? Sure you have. We all have. Consider my case in point. When I most needed a fast ride with qualified medics on board, I got not only one, but two. These men and women worked feverishly, and I'll never look at

another ambulance, EMT, firefighter, or police officer
the same way ever again.

At 9:06 p.m. the ambulance was en route to the first
of two hospitals I would visit before the crack of dawn
ever peeked over the horizon.

# ALIVE ON ARRIVAL

*"God put Rainbows in the clouds so that each of us—in the dreariest and most dreaded moments—can see a possibility of hope."*

Maya Angelou

The following accounts were provided to me from family members, a host of friends, physicians, and medical records surpassing eight hundred pages. Most I have no memory of. Some, I do. Some are funny…most are sobering. I don't make light of this tragic medical malady, as it almost took my life both literally and figuratively speaking. On the contrary, my hope is that these documented accounts make each reader aware. There will be no apology for including much needed comic relief in this, a journal I began for therapeutic reasons.

Early on in my recovery, I was lost to the world. The thought of never laughing again almost destroyed me. I'm ecstatic about having regained the sense of humor I thought was forever lost.

Ultimately, the emergency personnel employed by American Medical Response (AMR), transported me to the nearest medical facility, which is approximately seven miles from our home. Upon arrival at 9:23 p.m., I began displaying yet another symptom of a brain injury.

"Combative" is how my chart was documented. Or as Joel would later inform Frances, "She is really mad and screaming about still being in a lot of pain." The vomiting continued and the pain worsened, though it didn't seem conceivable from the initial onset.

My youngest sister, Frances, met Joel at the hospital after receiving a call from Kyle. With two ambulances parked in front of our house, the neighbors had now begun to make their way outdoors to see what was going on. Jason and Justin lived across the street, two doors down and grew up with my boys. Justin called Kyle on his cell phone to let him know something was wrong at our house and told him about the ambulances. Since Kyle was at work and not sure how to respond, he called his Auntie Frances, who in turn called Joel. Right about the time she made this call, AMR was prepared to transport me to the nearest hospital, Northeast Methodist. Joel asked Frances to meet him there, fielded a call from Kyle, and made the same arrangement with our son.

I regained consciousness upon arrival and was still in an enormous amount of pain. The ER doctors advised my family they could not administer any medications until they knew what they were treating. Within the first hour, I was sent to radiology for a CT scan to verify the suspicion of a brain bleed, which turned out to be caused by a ruptured 3-millimeter aneurysm.

Joel went back to the waiting room to give Frances an update. "They think it might be an aneurysm," he reported.

As Joel's lip quivered, Frances reached out and touched his arm. She wanted more than anything to comfort him and assure him everything would be okay. She just wasn't sure. This much she did know:

"I have to see her. I have to see my sister," Frances pleaded.

He gave her the ER room number, and she walked down the corridor and into the treatment room just as nurses were preparing for one final procedure prior to transporting me to a different facility. Regrettably, the hospital I had initially arrived at was not equipped to handle brain trauma.

After Kyle arrived at the emergency room, Joel briefed him and asked him to go home. He wasn't trying to hide anything from our son; he just did not want Kyle to see his mother in this state.

As Frances stood by my side, I remained totally oblivious to my surroundings. She figured the nurses must have sedated me or that I had lost consciousness once again since I lay there with my eyes closed and unresponsive. Why then, she asked herself, was I jerking and thrashing around so?

In the next few minutes, the emergency room doctor would brief my family. I was starting to show signs of respiratory failure, so a breathing tube was inserted in my throat. Instinctively, most patients will try to pull these tubes out, and I was no exception. My hands would be secured to the gurney with "soft cuffs." Once this procedure was completed, we were ready for immediate departure.

So urgent was their assessment, Air Life was summoned; however, there were no helicopters available, as they were already all in flight with other emergencies. My condition was critical with the hour now just after midnight. Our options were painfully simple. Wait for a helicopter to become available or make the trip in another ambulance. Joel chose the latter, and by the grace of God, at this hour, there was minimal traffic heading westbound on Loop 410, which also happened to be undergoing a major highway expansion renovation.

American Medical Response would once again be dispatched to transport me from one hospital to the medical center, and again, fate would intervene. Remarkably, the same two medics who transported me to the first hospital, Valerie Martinez and Dena Spring, received the dispatch call to transport me again. They truly understood the urgency, having witnessed firsthand my symptoms and having now been made aware of my diagnosis.

Frances listened as she was told where I was being taken and given instructions on how she should follow in her van. Law mandates vehicles remain fifty feet behind an ambulance in transport, which is evident by the speed, flashing lights, and sirens blaring. Both she and Joel would make their way to the Methodist hospital, centrally located in the heart of San Antonio's medical center.

The ambulance arrived at Methodist Medical Center, another seventeen miles away, at 1:37 a.m. Since the CT scans had already been electronically forwarded to their emergency room, a team assigned to my care was awaiting my arrival. Dr. Donald Hilton, the first of my two neurosurgeons, had a plan.

# HOME AWAY FROM HOME

*"When it looked like the sun wasn't going to shine anymore, there's a rainbow in the clouds."*

Maya Angelou

Joel made a call to his mother, and Frances was assigned the grim task of calling the rest of the family, including my out-of-state sister and already fragile father. Dad had not yet fully recovered from his quadruple bypass surgery the year before. When Frances made the call to Toni in Illinois at 1:00 a.m., Toni's heart sank. Middle-of-the-night phone calls rarely bring good news. Toni immediately thought this was the call she had always dreaded, the call reporting Dad's demise. "Are you awake?" Frances asked. "I need for you to be totally awake." She reassured Toni that dad was fine.

She barely had time to catch her breath when Frances told her, "It's Mickey, and it's really bad."

After briefing Toni with as much information as she had obtained, they debated about whether or not to call our father. Between Joel and the two sisters, they unanimously agreed he had to be informed, as devastating as it would be for him to learn. Toni offered to make the call, breaking the news to him as gently as possible, and would wait until she arrived the following day to give him all the details. It was in his best interest that he be kept somewhat sheltered for the immediate time being. Once they were off the phone, she would then proceed to get online and find the first flight to San Antonio that would depart O'Hare at daybreak.

A sense of urgency became evident as Dr. Hilton searched for someone to provide consent for the emergency surgery he needed to perform. The bleed was applying pressure on my brain, which could have serious consequences. Joel was still en route to the hospital as Frances continued her attempt to reach him on his cell phone. The calls appeared to be going through. However, because she was using her cell phone in the sub-level of the hospital, the calls dropped, one after the other. Just as Dr. Hilton was about to take it upon himself to sign the release, Frances got through to Joel, who gave his consent over the phone. He was minutes away from the hospital, but the procedure could not wait for him to arrive.

On his way to the operating room, Dr. Hilton stopped to address Frances. His compassionate demeanor comforted her, as he squeezed her shoulder and told her, "I am so sorry this is happening to your family. What has happened could take her life. We are going to do everything we can to save her."

Frances's reply was a simple plea. "No, we can't lose her. She's my world."

Shortly thereafter I would undergo the first of three brain surgeries. Dr. Hilton would perform the emergency ventriculostomy, a procedure that entailed having a burr hole, about the size of a common button, drilled into the back of my head. A tube was then inserted to drain the blood and fluid causing pressure on the brain. Closely monitored by a team of neurological professionals, we would wait and see.

To this day Frances claims there was something about Dr. Hilton's presence and compassion that brought her peace. He was most certainly instrumental in saving my life, and yet, I cannot remember him. In shear disbelief, Frances can't grasp this.

"When he checked in on you after your procedure, you were carrying on a conversation with him!" she exclaims. "You asked him if you were going to be able to make your trip to New York for your awards ceremony. Don't you remember? We all just exchanged glances with each other, up until he politely told you 'no'."

What she finds unbelievable, I find incredible. The inability to remember much of what happened and the weeks that followed would plague me for months.

Following this surgery I was taken to the Neurology Intensive Care Unit (NICU), where a diligent team of nurses would oversee my care. Multiple intravenous lines had been inserted in both arms and both hands to administer constant medications. Frances and Joel watched as a constant flurry of activity took place over my bed. To prevent the danger of further vomiting while intubated, a nurse pumped my stomach of any remains that hadn't already been expelled in earlier episodes. Some things are best not remembered.

Eventually Frances encouraged Joel to go home and check on Kyle, eat, secure the house, and try to get some sleep.

Although my eyes would open and close, I was not lucid or coherent. My baby sister waited quietly by my side, dozing for a few minutes at a time by resting her arms and head on the bedside table. At 5:30 a.m. the following morning, Frances woke up to a figure standing in the doorway of my room.

Dad had arrived and stood leaning in the doorway, as he could not bring himself to my bedside. Frances got up and walked over to hug and kiss him. They stood silently for a few minutes, and then, holding his hand, she guided him to my bed.

"Aye pobre mija" (oh, my poor baby/daughter), he cried.

She updated him on my progress, procedures, and prognosis. He had not slept all night, drove himself across town to the hospital, and was now beginning to display symptoms of anxiety combined with fatigue.

He began trembling, so after a brief visit, Frances walked him back to his vehicle and sent him home to eat and rest. Had this brief visit done him more harm than good?

"I would have crawled across town on my hands and knees to be by your side," Dad would later tell me. The love of a parent cannot be measured.

In the midst of the chaos, Frances also had the insight to remember to call my employer to notify them of this unexpected development. She knew my director, Charlotte Aaron, but didn't have her cell phone number. In the early hours of Sunday morning, Frances would need to get resourceful to make this connection prior to Monday morning, when I would be expected at the office.

Luci has been a personal friend and coworker for a better part of the twenty-seven years we've known each other. Back in 1985, we were even roommates for a while. At the time, we were both single parents of three-year-old boys, born three weeks apart from each other. She is the type of person who will show up at a hospital waiting room with tacos and snacks to feed your family because she knows they would not leave your side. In fact, she did indeed arrive at the hospital, shortly after she received the call from Frances, with tacos, snacks, *and* blankets. Again, she anticipated someone might be cold, sitting in the waiting room for extended periods of time.

Whenever I encounter, hear about, or read about some really awful person, I stop and reflect upon the

remarkable acts of kindness I have been blessed to be
on the receiving end of. There are far more good deeds
than bad. Again, I thank God for my everyday blessings.

Frances called Luci somewhere around 6:30 a.m.
on Sunday. Luci, the early-bird that she is, was
already awake and busy doing things around her
house. She would later tell me the news caught her
totally off guard.

"I was hearing everything Frances said, but it just
didn't seem real. I had just seen you at work the Friday
before, and you were fine. 'How could something like
this be happening,' was all I could think," Luci would
share with me over dinner much later.

Luci would provide Frances with Charlotte's phone
number, and then begin calling the rest of my "family" from work. Karen, Becky, Charlotte, Roxanne, Liz,
and Mando now joined Luci with the rest of my family
in the waiting room. By now, my mother; mother-in-
law; sister Lizz and her husband, Jake; and my brother,
Eli, had also arrived. Everyone was provided what
little news was available, which was essentially that I
had survived the surgery and remained in critical, but
stable condition.

Not wanting to impose, my coworkers headed to the
parking lot to hold their own vigil. Joel was touched by
the many visitors; however, he soon became weary of
all the commotion and asked that visitors be limited to
our immediate family members. He understood everyone meant well; he just wasn't able to accommodate

and focus on everything that was happening with me at the same time.

While Frances tried to keep everyone updated, she had not yet had her moment of reckoning. Once Mom arrived, Frances was no longer able to keep her composure. She embraced Mom and cried. She cried hard and for many reasons. She feared for my prognosis, she was overwhelmed by Luci's kind gestures, and was eternally grateful for the support shown by the multitude of friends who arrived so early that morning. Finally, when Becky informed her she had called her brother, a missionary in Africa, and asked him to put me on their prayer list, she could no longer hold back her tears. By now they were happy tears, as she felt promise with all that was happening. It wouldn't be long before I was on the prayer lists of family, friends, and strangers alike. The power of prayer would prevail.

When Mom tried to send a now exhausted Frances home to get some rest, she adamantly refused. She did, however, leave briefly that Sunday afternoon to pick Toni up from the airport. They both immediately returned to the hospital where Toni saw first hand her oldest sister laden with intravenous lines; partially shaved head, breathing tube down her throat, and a bit unkempt. These sisters began to ask the nurses tons of questions and get permission to clean me up a bit. They both understood the nurses had far more critical issues to contend with regarding my care, so they asked if they could scrub the iodine off the side of my face and neck, clean the residual vomit they could see up my nostrils, and remove what little make-up that was smeared over my face. While Joel went downstairs for coffee, the Antu sisters got busy.

When Frances finally went home late Sunday night, Toni and Joel remained by my side. When Joel headed home to feed the dog, check up on Kyle, shower, and secure the house, Toni stayed at the hospital. Between the three of them, I was only alone when taken away for procedures such as CT scans, angiograms, and surgery. There would always be at least one family member present at the hospital.

On Monday, two days after the rupture, I was breathing well enough on my own to have the breathing apparatus removed. The nurse explained the extubation process—how this tube would be removed, what to expect afterward—and pleaded for me to remain silent for at least one hour. I acknowledged her request by nodding my head up and down. No talking for one whole hour. Although Frances said the removal process looked absolutely horrible, not to mention painful, the device was removed without incident. Again, I have no recollection and cannot imagine sitting still for this. At best, it could be said that I was described as "loopy" a good part of the time, which should come as no surprise, given the volume of medications I was receiving. True to my word, I didn't speak...until the nurse exited my room.

As soon as she was out of earshot, I spoke, and will forever be ashamed of the very first words that came out of my mouth.

"Did somebody call my work?" I asked.

Both Toni and Frances responded, "Yes," and reminded me I shouldn't be talking.

"Does daddy know?" I asked immediately thereafter, ignoring their warning.

Again, they both assured me that everything had been taken care of, everyone had been notified, and finally pleaded with me to stop talking.

For now, although I was still listed as "critical," things were starting to look promising. No one could anticipate how this was going to change in a few short hours.

The following day, early morning on Tuesday, March 4, I began experiencing pain again. Intense pain, and this time it was different. I understood what was happening now and was very scared.

Once an aneurysm has ruptured, there is a good chance it will clot itself off to prevent any further damage, until damage control can be implemented. Another trip to radiology for yet another CT scan revealed instead continued bleeding on the brain. This is a pain that cannot be reasoned with. It was a diabolical condition that had to be corrected.

Dr. Vardiman would arrange for this to happen. After a thorough visit to discuss our options—which turned out to be very limited—and answer all of our questions, he scheduled the surgery to clip the aneurysm. A nurse would assist with the signing of multiple consent forms, and I was prepared to undergo my second brain surgery in three days. While in the holding area, I continued to be afraid. Only two family members are permitted to wait with you in this area, so Joel remained while Toni and Frances took turns coming in and out. It was only a matter of time before they decided they would both stay until one of them was asked to leave. Frances monitored my facial expressions, and I repeatedly cried, "It hurts!"

Within the half hour, Dr. Vardiman returned to my bed, looked at each of my family members, and boldly asked, "Do you mind if we say a prayer?" Without hesitation everyone took the hand of the person standing next to him or her. Dr. Vardiman prayed. It was a beautiful, eloquent prayer, administered by none other than a very humble neurosurgeon. A gifted surgeon who perhaps recognized he was not able to perform these procedures without divine guidance. When he concluded the prayer, he informed us he was headed to the operating room, where I would follow shortly thereafter. He walked away, and Joel and Frances felt a sense of calmness and panic at the same time.

So extraordinary was this gesture, they couldn't help but to wonder if this was some sort of preliminary "last rites" that was being administered. Why is it that when we most need to rely on our faith, we oftentimes find ourselves questioning solid ground?

Once I had arrived in the bright white, sterile operating room, calmness swept over me. "You are in good hands, and God has a plan," I kept reminding myself. God has a plan. This would become my credo. Again, even when there might have been a shred of doubt, I knew God had a plan.

This visit to the O.R. would entail a full-blown right frontotemporal pterional craniotomy, a right anterior temporal lobectomy, and the clip obliteration of complex right middle cerebral artery aneurysm. Finally, for this round, the microplate fixation of my skull flap. A detailed report chronicles this procedure as follows:

> After the controlled induction of general anesthesia, multiple large bore IV access, Foley catheter, TED pneumatic hose secured. The patient was positioned supine, head fixed in the Mayfield three-point fixation and a shave, prep, and drape of the right frontotemporal region was accomplished.
>
> A 10-blade knife was used to incise just anterior to the tragus from anteriorly to superiorly to midline and the myocutaneous flap rolled anteriorly over a rolled moist Raytech sponge with fish hooks used to maintain bony exposure. Calvarial perforation was accomplished with the high speed air drill and completed with a plated B1 attachment, bringing our dissection flush with the anterior adrenal fossa using high speed air drill and Leksell and double action rongeurs.
>
> A durotomy was performed with a 15-blade knife and scissors and the dura was done with the 4-0 Nurolon sutures. The ventriculostomy catheter remained in place with simple dissection to allow egress of spinal fluid. The brain was full to the point of being a danger in terms of potential pressure risks and a right anterior

temporal lobectomy was accomplished, allowing further egress of the spinal fluid through the temporal horn as well as brain relaxation, which allowed for a pulsatile slack brain through the procedure.

Under direct microsurgical visualization, the right middle cerebral artery aneurysm was identified with proximal and distal vasculature identified. A small bayoneted Yasergill straight clip was utilized to obliterate the intradural aneurysm preserving afferent and efferent vasculature and reconstructing the afferent vessel which was incorporating the aneurysm.

After copious irrigation and meticulous hemostasis, the wound was closed in a water-tight fashion with 4-0 Nurolon suture. Osteomed plating system was used to replace the bone flap and the temporalis and galea were closed with 2-0 Vicryl suture and sterile stainless steel staples. The ventricular catheter was reattached to a sealed drainage system. The patient was returned to the intensive care unit.

In just two hours Dr. Vardiman removed a section of my skull measuring approximately the size of a half-dollar to reach the 4-millimeter aneurysm that needed to be clipped. Clipping is the process of using a tiny, clothespin-like titanium clip to obliterate the aneurysm. Once clipped, blood no longer enters the aneurysm, which eliminates future bleeding. This procedure protects nearby brain tissue from further damage.

Dr. Arnold B. Vardiman will forever be one of my very own personal heroes. How can you *not* admire a man who opens up your head not once, but twice, and puts you back together, has witnessed blood flowing freely throughout your brain, would move heaven and earth to bring you back as the same person you had all but departed as?

No, I never saw that proverbial "light" we have all heard about. Nor did I hear anyone tell me to "go into the light." Even if I had, I'm certain Doc would have said, "Not on my watch she won't."

Running scared, my family would place my fate in God's hands. They understood Dr. Vardiman's own skilled hands were a gift, and they prayed and rallied for him as he performed such an intricate procedure, soon to be followed by another. These hands would repair damage not yet fully understood by mere mortals. The outcome would not have been successful if not for the passion of a doctor and faith that was growing by the minute.

Remember, God puts the right people, in the right place, at the right time.

Every now and then I awoke to someone standing at the side of my bed. Toni and Frances I remember. Regretfully, I don't recall my boys or my beloved dad. I vaguely remember Joel, and he spent most of his waking hours at the hospital. I certainly don't recall his dictating who was and was not allowed to visit, and I don't remember his constant partnering with my nursing team. In reality, my recollection of most of my hospital stay is patchy at best. Dr. Vardiman assured me this is a common phenomenon for patients following a brain hemorrhage, surgery, and a lengthy hospital stay.

Then suddenly someone I knew and recognized would appear at my bedside, but I wasn't quite sure why *he* or *she* was there. This couldn't be good. These were people from my past, extended and, sometimes, distant family members who were randomly showing up at my bedside. Were they saying their good-byes? Did I really see them? Either way, the odds did not appear to be in my favor.

One of the bigger challenges while in the NICU after the initial ventriculostomy was being instructed to remain still, very still. Keep in mind that I was kept pain-free in terms of medication, so surgical pain was not an issue. Simply put, I had been positioned in a semi-elevated position in my hospital bed, with a laser device aimed at the side of my head that would regulate the drainage of blood and CSF (cerebral spinal fluid) into an IV bag. Reverse osmosis, if you will. Maybe it was just me, but being told I couldn't move suddenly made me want to do anything and everything other than remain still. This quickly became a challenge my nursing team and family members would need to contend with, pretty much around the clock. If I wasn't sleeping, I was bored, and if I was bored, well, you can pretty much guess where I'm going with this.

Rumor has it, I did everything I was asked not to do: elevate the bed, lower the bed, ask for a phone, beg for a phone, and call my office.

Yes, although I have no memory of doing so, I'm told by reliable sources that I not only called my office once but managed to access a phone and call three times! Another medical marvel.

As the story goes, I kept getting on the phone to check on work. Joel had the phone in my room removed, so I began to borrow cell phones. As long as someone would accommodate me with a phone, I called my office. Charlotte called Joel to give him a heads up. He in turn had a talk with the director of nurses. Under no circumstances should I be given a phone. Period. The last young man I asked to borrow a phone from immediately disappeared and was not seen again. Word had indeed circulated—no phone calls.

Besides, how can someone be bleeding into her brain and yet still have the ability to remember incomplete projects sitting on her desk with deadlines imminently approaching? My nursing team was extremely compassionate and each had the "patience of the biblical Job."

If and when push came to shove, and for my own safety, restraints were used. Soft, white mitts covered my hands, and soft straps secured my wrists to the bedrails.

After my dad's open-heart surgery, he too lay in the ICU restrained in this same fashion. It broke my heart to see him this way, even though I understood what necessitated it. I prayed my boys hadn't seen me this way, and if they had, I hoped they too understand why this had to be. The last thing anyone needed was for me to suffer a fall or yank the catheter out of my head.

Although the drainage eventually yielded very little blood, there was still too much cerebral spinal fluid in my head. Hydrocephalus was the byproduct of my sub-arachnoid hemorrhage. Excessive CSF had no outlet and would begin to accumulate within the ventricles of my brain. Another medical intervention was about to take place. Ten days after the aneurysm rupture and first major surgery, I was back in the operating room to have a permanent shunt implanted on the oppo-site side of my head. With this newfound revelation, I opted to have the rest of my hair completely shaved off. The first two surgeries had already warranted for most of the right side of my head to be shaved. I couldn't imagine seeing myself half shaved on one side and a small section of hair shaved from the other side.

"Let's just shave what's left of my hair now and let it all grow back at the same time," I rationalized with the nurse. She, in turn, informed me we would need to obtain Dr. Vardiman's consent to shave my head.

"Why? He doesn't need my consent to get his hair cut," I would argue.

While awaiting Dr. Vardiman in the pre-op area, Frances and I were making small talk with the nurses. Sure enough, Doc came strolling over to my holding area, and I got my first good look at him—while in a rare, lucid state of mind. As one might imagine, I can't recall much of what was going on the first several days I was in NICU. It may have been the temporary induced coma or the massive amounts of medications, but I have very little recollection of any of the dozens of doctors at my bedside at any given time. On the contrary, according to my medical records, it appears there were doctors in and out of my room day and night.

Suffice it to say, when I did see this doctor approach my bed and heard the nurse address him as Dr. Vardiman, I just had to say, "Please tell me you graduated in the top 5 percent of your class."

Frances swears this was *the* defining moment for her. The moment when she was certain I was still "Mickey." She can't honestly say she was appalled by my query. This was comic relief, and I've used it all my life. What prompted me to ask Doc this very silly, personal, if not inappropriate question? I'll tell you why. It was because he appeared to be about twenty-five years old. *Wonderful*, I thought. *In my most desperate hour, I have "Doogie Howser" taking care of me.*

He played along. "I assure you, I did much better than 5 percent," he replied. Doc gave his consent for a complete shave, and, shortly thereafter, I was given that infamous injection of "top shelf" into my intravenous line. Clippers were taken to my head, working around the six-inch incision that had been made days before. I would undergo a smaller incision this time around.

Thursday, March 13, I would undergo my final surgical procedure. With a diagnosis of Post Hemorrhagic Hydrocephalus, came the placement of a left frontoventricular canal shunt. Detailed operative report as follows:

> The patient was brought to the operating theater and after controlled induction of general anesthesia, shave, meticulous prep and drape of the scalp was undertaken. Anterior cervical abdominal and chest wall regions were prepped and draped as well. A #10 blade was used to incise the skin with the muscle splitting exposure in the right upper quadrant, exposing the peritoneal contents. A single curvilinear perforation was made in the frontal region allowing for atraumatic placement of a ventricular catheter in the left frontal horn and allowing for placement of the subdermal tubing. Peritoneal catheter and appropriately oriented valve mechanism, which was secured to the ventricular catheter, slow cerebrospinal fluid, these were drawn, skin surface. Spontaneous flows demonstrated that the peritoneal cavity was placed under direct visualization into the peritoneal cavity. After copious irrigation and meticulous hemostasis, the wound was closed with #2-0 Vicryl suture, sterile stainless steel skin staples. Previously placed ventriculostomy catheter was carefully withdrawn following the procedure.

What the heck? Could this be normal? Yes, it was. One end of a tube was inserted into a ventricle, and the other end snaked all the way down the side of my head, down the inside of my neck and down to the peritoneal cavity, where the CSF would be deposited. The excess fluid would be absorbed into my bloodstream. Did you ever find yourself questioning your doctor? As in, he can't possibly know what he's talking about or contemplating doing? Yeah, I sell advertising for a living, and I am going to question my brain surgeon. Whatever.

The shunt implant procedure went well, and I would find myself back in the NICU for another five days. Surprisingly, I felt no discomfort from either of the incisions on top of my head. Headaches were tolerable. The incision made on my abdomen, however, had me utilizing my self-medicating pump as often as was regulated. I actually hit the button every few seconds, but was only administered as much morphine as was allowed.

As much as I begged, cried, and bribed, I was not allowed out of bed. I had now been mostly confined to bed for over two weeks and my body ached from top to bottom. If I made any attempt to re-position myself, in which case I'd more often than not make some groaning sound, there was always a nurse standing by to administer more pain medication. I wasn't in that kind of pain, but let's just say, they were very generous with the pain meds. Comfort and well-being was a huge mission of this neuro team.

I ate in my bed, was occasionally restrained to my bed, and eventually, bathed in that very same bed.

Who knew? One day a very sweet nurse approached me and asked if I'd like to have a bath. Yes! I was going to get out of the bed! I can only imagine the look of disappointment on my face when she informed me she would be bathing me *in* my bed. *Oh, a sponge bath*, I thought, as I rolled my eyes. No, it turned out she really bathed me. A full-fledged bath, with bins of water, soap, wash cloths, etc. By the time she was done, I was squeaky clean, dried off, and dusted with baby powder.

Washing my hair, or lack thereof, was not an issue.

Not that I wasn't grateful to be finally getting cleaned up a bit, but I would much rather have raced her down the hall to a shower/bathtub facility for a bona-fide, scalding hot water shower or bath! This wasn't going to happen anytime soon. These nurses really frowned upon patients running up and down the corridors of this intensive care unit.

Now that the sheets were soaking wet, surely I would be able to get out of this bed. What would we do? Before I could even begin to process how this dilemma would be resolved, she re-appears with a stack of clean linens. Yes, I was going to get out of the bed! Nope, it still wasn't going to happen today. It was apparent the medical professionals have learned many a trick-of-their-trade when a patient must remain confined to bed. She proceeded to roll me on my side in one direction and lift the sheets off the bed. Going around my bed, she rolls me in the opposite direction and, *viola*! She removed the sheets from that side, and I'm now lying on a bare, plastic covered mattress. Yes, I was going to…no, I wasn't getting out of bed. I should have seen that coming. She proceeded to put clean, dry sheets on the same way she took the wet sheets off. Roll, place, tuck. Roll, place, tuck. Pure genius.

A surprise visitor came one afternoon in the form of a reddish-blonde, four-legged therapy dog by the name of Botcke. She was accompanied by her two handlers and was the sweetest creature I'd ever seen. A large breed, she appeared to be an Irish Setter mix. This was not a figment of my imagination or a drug-induced hallucination. Joel was there, and he saw the dog too! You might think there are policies prohibiting dogs in an intensive care unit, but I was thrilled and had absolutely no objection. Research shows animals are capable of providing therapeutic, healing powers! Petting a dog can lower blood pressure, and who doesn't love a dog wearing a "Therapy/Service Animal" vest? One of Botcke's handlers provided me with some kibble to offer this extremely disciplined and remarkably trained service dog. I fed this beautiful beast one kibble at a time, in an attempt to stretch our visit. I didn't want to see her leave, but she had more patients to visit. You could tell this was her calling, her passion. Months later it would occur to me that during this poignant canine visit, I had no recollection of my own beloved Tobias "Pup"-odopolous. Toby was a rescue Joel and I adopted during the 2004 Summer Olympics, held in, where else, Athens, Greece.

The first time my feet touched the floor was several days later when a nurse wanted me to go "poo." What? Was I three years old now? Hey, if this was what it would take, I would gladly accept the proposal. I couldn't however, go to a private bathroom. I'd have to use a mobile potty chair positioned next to my bed—assisted and monitored no less. Pardon *moi*? I guess the hospital didn't want to be held liable for any pain-killer-induced patient falling off a commode and breaking anything else of value. I knew I must have been making some healing progress because I was getting pretty agitated by now. I had a hard enough time using a public restroom (with a door that closed) and was now asked to go behind a curtain? If we could establish all my "plumbing" was working, I could leave NICU and head down to a private room on the ninth floor. Now that was incentive enough for me. I became gung-ho. Besides, surely I wasn't the first person they'd ever seen go "poo," right?

Embarrassing as this was, it finally happened, and I was given my walking papers, so to say. Shortly before 9:00 p.m., I was transferred to the general population neuro ward on the ninth floor. My very own room, complete with a shower, a toilet, and a door for privacy! Since visiting hours were over, Joel had already left the premises. This meant I would be relocated to my private room unaccompanied. I now had the liberty to roam the halls as often as I liked, raise and lower my bed all I wanted, and shower as often as I liked for the duration of my stay.

What I hadn't done for the two weeks I had been in NICU was see my image in a mirror. It was now time to see what all the commotion was about. Time to see why whenever a visitor approached for the first time, their eyes would tend to involuntarily widen.

Slowly, like a ninja in the night, I approached the bathroom. As I turned the corner to face the mirror, there was a strange sensation hanging over me. Was someone standing there? The person I had briefly seen in the mirror could not have possibly been that of my own reflection. Turning around quickly, I realized there was no one else in the room. I was alone. After much hesitation, I slowly looked back into the mirror and stared. Without moving, I remained fixated for several minutes. Tears began filling my eyes. There was no way to be prepared for what I witnessed.

No hair. Pale, pasty-looking complexion, with slightly blackened eyes. Fresh incisions held together by dozens of staples on both sides of my head. The right side displayed an indentation, while the left side displayed a huge knot, which is the shunt that sat directly underneath my scalp. I closed my eyes and heard myself speak out loud. "God, please don't let babies be afraid of me," I prayed.

For the first time in the two weeks I had now been in the hospital, I was alone and inconsolable. Suddenly exhausted, I went back to my bed and sat down. My niece Skylar was only six months and my goddaughter Leah was a toddler of three years. I adore these girls and couldn't help but to think they might pull away in fear if I reached for them. My heart ached.

Skylar would soon put this fear to rest when she arrived with her mom for a visit a couple of days later.

As I lay in bed, I held my arms out to her, and she immediately came to me. I cried. She did not.

It would purposely be another three months before I saw Leah. As she was a bit older, I wanted to heal a bit and try to bear some resemblance to myself before our first encounter. I just didn't want her to be afraid. Turns out, she was as resilient as Sky. She would run up to me, wrap her little arms around my legs and yell "Nina!" Again, I cried, and she didn't. Crying would become a mainstay of my life for the next four months.

If I wasn't already terribly self-conscious about my appearance, things were going to get worse. Only this time, I would find humor in my "battle scars." Lying in my hospital bed one afternoon, I was determined to try and remove the surgical tape that attached a monitoring device on my finger. An oxygen-level monitoring device, if memory serves me right. After a few minutes of pulling and tugging, I decided to use my teeth. Yes, I was about to do something I preached to my sons *not* to do. All I needed was a good grip on the tape, and I would give it a hard yank. Almost immediately, I heard something hit the floor with a *clink*. Looking down at my finger only proved my attempt to chew the tape off was a complete failure. The monitor was still securely taped in place. Sitting up on the side of my bed, something felt peculiarly different inside my mouth. Now missing, was the crown that covered my front eyetooth! It would appear I no longer had my five-thousand-dollar-braces smile to compensate for the rest of these physical imperfections.

While staring in the mirror at the collateral damage I had done, what was that music I was hearing? Was it dueling banjos? Yes, without doubt, I could have auditioned for an extra on the set of a *Deliverance* remake, and would have won the part of one of those mountain folks hands-down.

My final week in the hospital was spent resting and healing. The nursing team was attentive, albeit less intrusive than the nurses in NICU who were constantly hovering around checking on one thing or another.

There was a steady stream of visitors now that I was settled in to a private room. Joel, Toni, and Frances were practically permanent fixtures. Kim, a long-time friend and masseuse, would come to the hospital to massage my legs, which had begun to cramp terribly. Potassium levels had dropped low enough to raise a red flag.

In between visits from family and friends, waking hours were spent walking up and down the long hallways of this ward. This was a relatively easy task since there was not a conventional IV pole to drag around. A "pic line" (central intravenous line) had been inserted into my neck early on, which allowed for the constant blood draws needed for various labs and the ongoing administration of intravenous medications.

As I walked these hallways, I felt remarkably strong and wondered what all the fuss was about. I still didn't have a clear understanding of what had happened to me or why. Simply put, I didn't grasp the severity of my condition. Since I felt minimal pain and was not experiencing any physical deficits, I did not, nor could I, comprehend.

The worst was yet to come.

Shortly before my discharge, a nurse came to talk to me about going to a rehabilitation facility. I would not be released to go directly home. The consensus was I would be discharged to a rehabilitative center for an additional week of observation and therapy.

Staring out of my hospital-room window, I yearned to be outdoors. It had now been the better part of the month of March since I had been hospitalized. There was a burning desire to feel the sun on my face and experience the cool spring breeze blowing about. Toni and Frances would make this happen. With permission granted from the nursing station and a wheelchair in tow, I took a seat, and we headed for the elevators. Excitement welled up within me to the point that I imagined we were all making the great getaway. I pounded on the "close-door" button to the elevator so we would no longer be visible in the event the nurse changed his mind.

My two accomplices would spend the next forty-five minutes taking turns pushing my wheelchair around the main entrance to the hospital. The sun was shining, the flowers were in full bloom, and birds were singing. It was indeed a glorious day. We found a place to park next to a bench, strategically located next to a newspaper vending machine. It was a Sunday afternoon. I was coherent enough to remember the paper should be publishing their 2008 Excellence & Leadership Award winners about this time.

The awards ceremony was held on February 17, at Sunset Station in downtown San Antonio. I was honored to have received one of two Marketing Excellence Awards, second only to the coveted Hearst Eagle Award. This would prove to be the grandest highlight of my twenty-four-year career with Hearst Corporation. Along with the recognition came a sizeable monetary bonus and an all-expense-paid trip to New York for a formal awards presentation ceremony. Winners would also be treated to a fabulous stay at the Essex Hotel, a Broadway show, tour of the newly completed Hearst Tower, and other fun-filled activities. I had never been to New York and was over-the-moon excited to have both won this prestigious award and also have the opportunity to see my former publisher, Mr. George Irish, who would present the awards at a special luncheon ceremony. Excited was an understatement. I would visit the Hearst Tower and everything else New York had to offer!

Frances purchased the paper from a nearby vending machine. Sure enough, there was the traditional full-page "circle-of-winners," complete with photos taken the night of the awards ceremony. Gingerly, I touched my photo. My fingers outlined what had been my hair only six weeks earlier. Yes, only six weeks earlier, when my life was normal.

Days after my discharge, word arrived the trip to New York was scheduled for May 30. I would not be strong enough by then, nor would I get a doctor's consent to travel so soon. Again, I would cry. Again, I would ask "why?"

March 19 was my release date from Methodist Medical Center. Although every experience I had at the hospital was one hundred and ten percent top notch, I was more than excited to be discharged and that much closer to getting home. As we waited for discharge orders, the removal of my central IV line, and the notorious wheelchair ride to my waiting vehicle, I squirmed with excitement. Again, there just wasn't a real clear picture of how serious this ordeal was or what lay ahead of me for the next several months. I felt fine at this point. Looked like a train-wreck, but I felt fine.

Joel drove me directly to the rehab facility, where I would be under observation for the next several days. Here, I would work with a physical therapist, occupational therapist, and speech therapist to ensure I was capable of caring for myself once I got home. Up until now, in light of all that had taken place in the last three weeks, my progress had been good. Within a matter of hours, this was once again going to change dramatically.

We arrived at the rehab center around 4:00 p.m. The staff was expecting my arrival, having coordinated with the nurses at the hospital. A nurse led us to my semi-private room and got me settled into bed. *Wonderful*, I thought. *They are going to put me straight to bed.* I was beginning to feel like a rebellious child by now. A curtain separated the double-occupancy room beds, and although I didn't know it at that very moment, my stay at this facility would be incredibly short.

Once situated, Joel departed to get me some "street" clothes and sneakers. Hospital gowns had made me a fashion victim for long enough. Besides, I needed apparel suitable for the physical therapy I would begin the following day. While I attempted to eat a very bad dinner, Joel drove to the nearest Wal-Mart to purchase these items. There was no sense in his driving all the way out to Converse and back again. Upon his return, he sat with me until visiting hours were over. The eerie feeling that had overcome me when we arrived earlier that day continued to plague me. Couldn't quite put my finger on it, but something was amiss. The night nurse allowed me to pace the halls, which I did for the better part of the night. Eventually I grew tired and returned to my room and bed and tried to sleep. I was aroused periodically to take meds and have my vitals assessed. At 5:00 a.m. I got out of bed, washed up, and got dressed. I was told to expect the first of my three therapists around 6:00 a.m. The occupational therapist was the first to arrive and was surprised to see me fully dressed, tennis shoes and socks included. She explained that she needed to watch me dress myself. I looked at her in disbelief. Two things crossed my mind in these wee hours of the morning. First, if she wanted to see me dress myself, she should have been at my room at 5:00 a.m. Second, who did she *think* dressed me? Trying extremely hard to understand her plight, I agreed to undress and get re-dressed while she cautiously observed. I finished by tying my shoes, and she seemed quite impressed. It took a minute for the realization to hit me. Not *everyone* is capable of doing these simple tasks following a brain injury. Now I felt guilty. If I had struggled, she would have assisted me. She would have taught me to dress myself again, if the need had presented itself. She proceeded to explain how she would chart my progress for the rehab doctor, who would be in to see me sometime around the lunch hour.

The physical therapist and speech therapist would arrive shortly to visit with me and make their own assessments.

Breakfast arrived around 7:30 a.m., and I found myself growing increasingly anxious. Although I understood the purpose of rehab, understood everything I was told, I suddenly decided I did not want to be there. I did not *need* to be there. My breakfast would have to wait. There was a plan I needed to outline and execute in the next couple of hours.

The physical therapist arrived around 9:00 a.m. After a few questions, we were headed toward the gymnasium. As I sat up to get off my bed, she prepared to wrap a gait belt around my waist. Again, I understood this was a safety precaution, but nonetheless, objected. I explained I had been walking up and down hospital corridors for many days by now and was steady on my feet. She obliged and asked that I take extreme caution and walk side by side with her. The gym was on the other side of the facility, and I followed her step for step. When the therapist opened the double door to the gym, I was overcome with sorrow.

A huge, open gym that housed many pieces of equipment was one hundred percent occupied. Every treadmill, stair-climber, exercise ball, and jump rope was in use. The only "tool" available was a man-made platform with five steps on either end. The therapist led me over and asked if I would be able to climb up and down these stairs a couple of times while we waited for some other piece of equipment to become available. I was able and climbed up the stairs and back down, twice. Then I asked if we could leave. She agreed we would come back later when the crowd thinned out. We returned to my room, and she would leave for the time being to file her report.

As soon as she left, I pressed the nurse-call button and requested that a nurse come to my room. While waiting for her, I called Joel and asked him to come and pick me up. Now. Right now. Not later, but now. Not next week, when I was expected to leave, but now. I wanted to go home, and I was prepared to do whatever it took to be in *my* house, in *my* bed, that night. Perhaps I was having an irrational moment, but the way I felt at that exact moment, I was prepared to walk out of the facility and not look back until I turned onto Pepper Trail and walked through my front door.

Poor Joel. I could tell by his tone that he was a bit confused by this new development. He begged me to stay put…he was on his way. The nurse walked in, and I explained to her I wanted to go home. Now. Not next week, not tomorrow, but now. When she asked why, I explained I didn't belong here. Sadness had overcome me with the realization that I was occupying a bed, taking up space and resources that someone else needed more. She compassionately explained I couldn't leave until the doctor saw me, and it would be his decision as to whether or not I could leave this early in the rehabilitation program. She agreed to page him and let him know of my concern.

Meanwhile, I would take my breakfast and spread the contents all around the plate. Since I wasn't hungry, my intention was to try to fool whoever was responsible for charting how much of each meal had been consumed.

Joel arrived within the hour, followed by Dr. Onghai. After an extended visit, he agreed to review the therapists' reports and let me go home if they proved favorable. The speech therapist had not yet done her assessment, so I would need to complete her testing for Dr. Onghai's review as well. These were primarily cognitive tests, about half of which I struggled with. Please! Calculate long math, without a calculator? I couldn't do this *before* my brain injury. What I did fail miserably, to my astonishment, was the memory skill sets. This activity was one I normally excelled at. The therapist assured me this was to be expected and, with practice, I should regain this functionality. After completing worksheets in which I tallied up the number of nickels, dimes, and pennies illustrated and identified the time reflected on an animated clock, I was done with the last of my tests.

Now we just needed interpretations, or the report card, from the respective therapists. For the first time in my life, I was hoping to be "Teacher's Pet," and also hoped they would provide some sort of sliding grade.

After review of all the assessments, and comfortable I could manage most functions by myself, Dr. Onghai ordered my discharge with strict instructions to follow up with both Doctors Vardiman and Wiesenthal.

Orders were given to remove a portion of the staples from the one side of my head. Prescriptions were prepared, and I got ready for my discharge. I sat rigidly still while staples from the right-hand side of my scalp were gingerly removed. The other side, along with those on my abdomen, would be removed at a yet-to-be-determined date at my neurosurgeon's office.

Finally we went over each of the prescriptions written for my discharge, to include the elusive and very expensive anti-seizure medication Nimotop. One of the nurses was kind enough to call various pharmacies to find out who might have it in stock. This prescription had to be picked up before we returned home, as I would need to take two pills every four hours for the next several days.

After we left the rehab facility, Joel drove to the pharmacy a short distance away. We walked straight back to the pharmacy while other patrons stared at a pitiful looking woman in her robe, house shoes, and whose head looked like it had gone through a plate glass door. I didn't mind. All I wanted was to get what I needed and head home. The partial order of forty-six pills cost $524.89, out-of-pocket, with insurance. On one of my good days, I would have interrogated the pharmacy tech until I was blue in the face. Tonight, however, we would pull out our debit card and pay for it. These days it was imperative that I choose my battles carefully. This was a battle to be fought at a later date.

# SCARED DOESN'T BEGIN TO COVER IT

*"You gain strength, courage and confidence by every experience in which you really stop to look fear in the face. You must do the thing which you think you cannot do."*

Eleanor Roosevelt

We pulled into our driveway on the evening of Thursday, March 20, the day before Good Friday. Surely this had to be a good omen. It felt a bit strange returning to my house after such an extended absence. Plus, we were on our own now, with no doctors or nurses at our disposal, and as much as I wanted this, it turned out there was a tiny bit of apprehension. With discharge orders and prescriptions littering our kitchen counter, it was time for me to fly solo. Well, solo with my co-pilot, Joel, by my side. He set the alarm on his phone to go off every four hours, prompting us it was time to take the most critical of these medications, the Nimotop. This course of treatment began while in the hospital and was to be taken, without fail, around-the-clock for twenty-nine days to prevent the possible onset of seizures. "Mickey, do *not* miss a dose of this medication. It is crucial that this medication be taken on schedule, without fail," my nurse pleaded. No pressure here.

Then there was the Dilantin, Vicodin, Azithromycin, Pantoprazole, Klor-Con, Diphenoxylate, Metronidazole, Gabapentin, yada, yada, yada.

What I wasn't receiving anymore was intravenous morphine. Didn't need it and didn't want it. Or so I thought. The pain I was experiencing was manageable, even without hardcore prescription medication. Someone forgot to tell this to the rest of my body. It had now gone without morphine for somewhere in the neighborhood of seventy-two hours.

The first night at home, in my own bed, would find me tossing and turning. Then I would begin to alternate between breaking into a sweat and then shivering as though I was freezing. What I initially thought was just a bad case of nerves turned out to be Morphine withdrawal. Now we would begin a regimen of meds to combat the withdrawal symptoms. *Brilliant*, I thought. As my goal was to try and narrow down the number of medications I would be taking, another prescription is called in.

A tracking system was desperately in order, so I would begin keeping a daily journal of when and which medications needed to be taken throughout the course of the day. It appeared to be non-stop.

Taking pills around the clock was a catch-22. The meds were doing what they were supposed to, however, consuming this volume of oral medication brought on its own set of issues: too much sleep, too much nausea, and eventually, too much insomnia. This pattern would repeat itself for several weeks. In my attempt to combat these issues, I had stopped eating.

It was no secret that I needed to lose weight; however, this was definitely not a recommended weight loss program. Effective, but not highly recommended. Three days later, on Easter Sunday, I ate for the first time since coming home. It was a beautiful day, and Joel grilled dinner for us and his mother, who arrived for a visit. The half-dozen bites of chicken fajitas I consumed would be the last I would eat for another two weeks. Talking to my mother-in-law would trigger the first of many meltdowns.

"Mom, I can't shake this eerie feeling. I have lost three weeks of my life, three weeks that I can't ever have back," I cried, as I referred to my injury and hospital stay, of which I could remember very little.

She would hug me then lean back and lovingly remind me of the reality of what was going on. "Mija, you didn't lose three weeks; you survived and have your whole life ahead of you," she enlightened me. This did bring me comfort, if only temporarily. Later it would become my mantra.

In the interim, my medications would continue to be monitored, altered, and taken religiously. Bottled water and sips of Ovaltine would become my staple for several weeks. Nothing was appetizing, and the pounds continued to drop. This was just one more thing to worry about. Drastic weight loss is never healthy, and I was creeping up on having lost thirty pounds in forty-five days. Joel was the first to observe as I turned down anything he offered to cook; refused any offer for take-out and had even given up my habitual three-plus cups of coffee every day. He worried, but he wouldn't give up. Every now and again and much to his delight, I would manage a bite or two. Without explanation some of my favorite foods would be permanently elim-inated, by choice, from my diet. Fried chicken, flour tortillas, and fried rice. Why? I simply didn't like them anymore. No one has been able to figure out why this happened, but my doctor reassures me I will survive just fine without these food choices. Go figure. Joel's theory is that my disdain for fried chicken is a mat-ter of "association." Fried chicken was the last thing I ate, only two hours prior to the rupture. We still can't explain the tortillas and fried rice. Perhaps someday the desire will return. Or maybe it won't. It is a strange phenomenon, but nothing to cause any harm or alarm. My passion for coffee did return after a few months.

I wanted nothing more than to have my old life back. It wasn't a perfect life, but I was happy with it just the way it was. Almost everything was now measured BA (before aneurysm) and AA (after aneurysm). Embracing my AA life would prove to be a work in progress.

Home for several days now, I finally decided to unpack my pink hospital tub, crammed full of all the little odds and ends you accumulate while in the hospital. Anything that was a reminder of my hospital stay went straight into the trash can: soap, toothpaste, shampoo, etc. Shampoo? Gait belt. Then I discovered a bundle of large four-by-four unwrapped gauzes. They felt thick, as though something was tucked away inside. Curious, I slowly unwrapped the layers of gauze until I came upon the contents. It took a few minutes for me to decipher exactly what it was I was staring at. Was it? It was! It was my signature big hair. My eyes filled with tears once again. Big, fat tears that would roll down my cheeks, fall onto, and bounce off the hardwood floor. I sat on the floor pondering. Someone actually took the time to gather my hair and pack it away nice and neat. Surely this someone had a true understanding of what a patient must feel when he or she discovers they no longer have their beloved mane. The compassion of this person, whoever he or she was, should not have gone unnoticed. If you are reading this passage, thank you.

I had already cried me a river the first time I saw my bald, bony "zipper-head" in that hospital room mirror. A zipper head is a reference made to an incision closed with staples, as it truly resembles a zipper. With this recollection, I threw the hair back in the tub and threw the entire tub in the trash can. Vanity plays no part in the attachment we have to our hair. It's hard to explain. A bad hair day is simply a bad hair day. A "no-hair" day takes on an entirely different meaning. The wonder of being bald grew on me, and I still think "bald is beautiful." You just need to get over the initial shock.

Once I had disposed of all these reminders, the smaller trash can was in turn hauled to the bigger trash can in the garage. If it had been remotely close to trash pick-up day, I would have pulled that can out to the curb right then and there. It's not that I wasn't appreciative of the Good Samaritan's intention. It's just that I didn't need or want any tangible reminders of my ordeal. Instead, I wanted to distance myself. I wanted all of these reminders out of my field of vision forever. I wanted to wish it had never happened. Just wish it away.

Within the next seventy-two hours, my body would begin to cease the "junkie" withdrawal symptoms and the long weaning process of numerous meds would be underway. Dr. Vardiman had already told me I would eventually be off all but the anti-seizure med, Dilantin. This medication would most likely need to be taken for the remainder of my life, to ward off any possible seizures. If this were the worst of what I was to endure, I would once again count my blessings.

The fear, however, would not leave me alone. The thought of being alone was petrifying, although that was my life before all of this. The sad reality was Joel had returned to work and Kyle was at school during the day and usually worked the 4:00 p.m. to 10:00 p.m. shift. If anything were to go wrong while home alone, I sincerely doubted that I would dodge the bullet a second time around. If not for the medications that were notorious for putting me to sleep, I would have been "eyes-wide-open" around the clock.

Then there was the *other* constant haunting.

Of all the bits and pieces of information that may have been permanently deleted from my "mainframe," one thought remained steadfast. What if Joel hadn't been home the night of the rupture? What if he had been at one of his Saturday night gigs that night? What if I had dropped to the floor and bled out. These weren't the thoughts that haunted me the most. It was this: If Joel *had* been at a gig, Kyle would have gotten home from work first. What if Kyle had found me? What if….

April 8 proved to be an unfortunate date in terms of setbacks. It had been barely two weeks since my release from the hospital, and although I had been feeling relatively well, an unexpected turn of events would soon unfold. Mid-morning found me lying on the bed in our guest room reading the paper. Tired of this resting, I would sit up in bed and immediately feel a sharp pain on my left side. Not yet concerned, I self-diagnosed a pulled muscle. I would simply "walk it off." Over the course of the next couple of days, the pain would become so intense, it became an effort to sit, stand, walk, get up, or get around at all. Absolutely perplexed, my primary care physician would write orders to admit me back to the Methodist hospital, conveniently located next to his office. There, I would undergo various tests to determine the cause of the pain and rule out any problems potentially related to my existing condition.

Upon learning of my re-admission, Dr. Vardiman, my neurosurgeon, checked in on me. I was concerned the left frontoventricular canal shunt tubing could somehow be causing this pain. CT scans ruled out this theory. Five days and several tests later, I was once again released from the hospital. The pain continued, while my walking around holding on to my left side became a familiar sight to everyone. Some days were worse than others, and there still appeared to be no rhyme or reason for the pain. As though I wasn't already consuming enough pills every day, one more would be added to assist with this pain management. Nerve damage? Probable. Most reassuring was the news that damaged nerves typically regenerate themselves.

# Rebuilding My Faith

*No vision, and you perish,*
*No ideal, and you're lost,*
*Your heart must ever cherish some*
*faith at any cost.*
*Some hope, some dream to cling to,*
*Some rainbow in the sky,*
*Some melody to sing to,*
*Some service that is high.*

Harriet Du Autermont

God knows I haven't *always* behaved like the Christian I know I am. Like everyone, I fall from His grace on occasion. I don't believe God *made* this happen to me, although He *allowed* it to happen and chose to spare me for a reason. For weeks, then months, I questioned "why?" Why me? I was scared, and then I was angry with myself for being so. Why did I survive when many don't? This was a constant reminder from well wishers who always shared stories of people they knew who had *not* survived a ruptured aneurysm. It seemed like every time I turned around, someone was telling me about the person they knew who "dropped dead" instantly from a ruptured aneurysm. They meant no harm and were truly amazed by my survival. Unfortunately, they didn't realize the implications of the comments made.

"Survivor's guilt" is defined as a mental condition that occurs when a person perceives himself or herself to have done wrong by surviving a traumatic illness or event that many others may not have survived. It's a miserable state of mind to reside in. I applaud every medical survivor, war hero, and every other type of survivor who has dealt with this demon.

My prayers became as regular as the days were long. I thanked God every time I woke up and every time I laid my head down to sleep again. I thanked Him for every one of my many doctors' appointments that showed continued progress. I thanked Him for my ability to walk, to talk, and to feed myself. But I still cried.

As the realization of my ordeal began to play itself out, the sheer beauty of His graciousness became very apparent to me. There was no room for argument. I am God's child and worthy of his ability to perform one of his many miracles on *me*—a modern-day miracle. We sometimes overlook these everyday blessings, unless they touch us this closely, this personally. Then, with the innocence of a child, we believe with every ounce of our being.

Joel was heaven-sent and a constant source of comfort. He is a big guy, and his massive chest became a resting ground for my face during my numerous, unpredictable meltdowns. Many a day he walked around wearing a tear-soaked T-shirt. Yes, God put him in my life for many reasons. I truly believe his presence at home on this fateful night was pre-conceived.

The Good Lord also gave Joel the strength to cope not only with me, but also with family, work, and friends…juggling all with what appeared to be effortless ability. How can you not believe? God has a plan, and I have complete faith in that.

Yes, every now and again, I get a pang in my head, and I panic. Is this a contradiction of my faith? Arguably, yes. The beauty is that He knows my heart, and I am, after all, human.

If you had told me that my life would return to any semblance of normalcy during the first four months following this aneurysm rupture, I would have called you a bald-faced liar. These were months of healing, overwhelming emotional turmoil, and daily struggle. It is said that "Laughter is the Best Medicine." Had I not been able to reach back into my past and retrieve the gift of humor, the healing process may have never come to fruition. Looking back, I said and did things that shocked many, me included.

# HELPING HANDS

*"Unless we think of others and do something for them, we miss one of the greatest sources of happiness."*

Ray Lyman Wilbur

One of the most amazing revelations during my recovery was that of all the prayer lists I had been placed on. Someone from this church then that church then another and another. Everyone I knew who attended church had placed me on his or her own church's prayer list. Absolutely incredible. Becky, a co-worker and long-time friend, immediately called her brother upon learning of my ordeal. A missionary stationed in Africa. Yes, I had people in Africa praying for me!

During the course of a long and ongoing recovery, family and friends provided me with much comfort and support. The daily phone calls, the visits, cards, flowers...all a constant reminder of how truly blessed I am. We can never forget how enriched our lives are by the presence of family and friends.

The day after my return home, I was compelled to make contact with my "kids" at work. A couple of my team members were a bit older than I, although most were younger and it was understood that as their manager, I considered them all my "charges." Our departmental administrative assistant, Denise, had done a remarkable job acting as the go-between with everyone at work. She constantly fielded questions from various colleagues at the paper, providing them with as much of an update as HIPAA would allow. Since she kept me abreast of all these inquisitions, I wanted to let my team know I was home and was doing as well as could be expected. I penned an open e-mail and happily awaited a stream of replies.

From: Mickey Urias
Sent: Friday, March 21, 2008 10:15 AM
To: Gregory, Carolyn; Laumer, Dennis; Graham, Diana; Urena, Dolores A; Moreno, Edward; Terrazas, Gilda; Viator, Jana; Alvarez, Jane; Muench, Matt; Sylvia Gartner; Starr, Lisa A; Southworth, April D; Pena, Michelle; Garza, Erik; Ybarra, Tanya M
Subject: Hello


Team,

Just a quick note to let you know I'm home and doing as well as can be expected. I busted out of rehab yesterday to get home to my family, as I hadn't seen Kyle in three weeks and was becoming inconsolable.

I just wanted to take the time to write you all and thank you so much for taking care of business in my absence. I've been in touch with Charlotte, and she has had nothing but good things to say about all you have accomplished. All that preaching to you all about the importance of teamwork was taken to heart and has made you guys shine! Keep up the good work, as you are all professionals at what you do. Continue to communicate with one another. Help each other out when needed, and your efforts and successes will not go unnoticed.

I can't say exactly when I will return to work, as my follow-up appointment isn't until next Friday, March 28th. I anticipate the doc will remove the bazillion staples in my head and on my belly; review the quadrillion medications I've been on (most temporary, I hope). I'm going to work on my rehab here at home, so hopefully I'll be getting stronger and fit. Just another quick warning...I don't have any hair, but hopefully it'll start growing back here pretty fast. I can't look in the mirror without crying...I don't know the person looking back. Okay, enough gloom and doom. Please continue doing what you have been...I can't express enough how proud of you all I am. Not to mention, it has taken a load off my worries that all is going smooth at the office. When the time is right, I will drop by to see you all. You are all certainly missed.

Until then, my sincerest thanks....
Mickey

P.S. If I missed anyone on the team, would someone please forward this e-mail to them? I stared at my distribution list for ten minutes, but for some reason, my memory isn't as sharp as it once was. J/K & LOL.

---

Mickey, I was so happy to read your email, we are all so glad that you are home. Please take care of yourself and do what you need to do so you can get back to us, we all miss you very much. Especially me. Your office is very lonely & quiet without you. Everyone here is fine, it's been a little slow this week w/Spring Break & *Easter* but we are chugging along like the little freight train. Please feel free to email or call me anytime you want and when you feel up to it I would love to come see you. Maybe your hair will come back curly (my grandmother's did). I bet Kyle is relieved that you are home. Have a Happy Easter!!!! I love you!

Jana Viator
Commercial Merchandise Rep

HEY YOU!!! We really do miss you too! We are so happy that you are doing so much better! Get plenty of rest Girlie!! Don't worry about us. You trained us very well. Have a very HAPPY EASTER!!! We missed you for St Patrick's Day! Kiley & I pray for you every night. I really do miss your GOOD MORNING EVERY-ONE!! Tell Joel thank you for taking care of you. We are so glad that he has been there for you. I am so glad that Kyle can see you again. I would like to visit you when you get better. I really miss you! You are the reason that I go so strong here! It brought tears to my eyes & now it is too to hear about this happening to someone that means the world to us! I put your photo of you on your wall of your office. It's the photo of you from the 2007 Awards. You look so adorable. Don't worry about your hair it will come back. You are beautiful in & out!

Lisa Anne Starr
Primetime Advertising Representative

MICKEY...I WANT TO SEE YOU...I MISS YOUR GOOD MORNING EVERYBODY AND I MISS YOU SO MUCH.... YOU DON'T EVEN KNOW HOW MUCH WE MISS YOU...BUT...YOU GET WELL AND REST ENOUGH TO GET SO WELL. YOU KNOW

YOU ARE BEAUTIFUL WITH HAIR OR WITHOUT....PLEASE KEEP IN TOUCH AS WE MISS THOSE EMAILS.. WHEN I FIRST SAW AN EMAIL FROM YOU MY HEART WAS HAPPY!!!!!!!!!!!!!!!!! !!!!!!!!!!!

LUV YOU & MISS YOU...ALL OF US DO....

GET WELL SOON...GOD BLESS YOU & YOUR FAMILY

Dolores A. Urena,
Commercial Advertising Representative

Mic,

How wonderful it is to hear from you and to know how well you are recovering!!! Please, please, please do not worry about anything here at the office. We all miss you terribly but we don't want you back until it's time....and then some. Don't rush coming back.....we're fine.

Before you know it...you'll have hair again. Hair or no hair you're still beautiful to everyone!! I don't know if you have a natural curl but all the people I've know that has gone thru this.....their hair has come back curly. Go figure!!!!

I'll cut this short cause I know you'll be receiving a lot of e-mails.....don't tire yourself & try to read them all at once. Just rest, rest, rest & let everyone pamper you.

> We'll see you when we see you.
> God Bless You Always!!!
> Love You!!!!!
> Gilda

---

Mickey,

You have no idea how relieved I am to be able to read this email from you. I just thank God you made it through this with the blessing of a recovery period ahead of you; it could have been so much worse. We may be doing okay without you, but your not being here with us makes a big difference. We feel your absence, and look forward to having you with us again.

Take care and let us hear from you. Know you are the "heart beat" of this team.

Carolyn

———————

Hello Mickey,

I am sorry it has taken me awhile to e-mail you back. I want you to know that we think about you here on a daily basis and I am glad that you are recovering so well. We do miss you here and we will be so excited for your visit. However, don't worry about us and take your time. Your job right now is to get well. Have you gone to any follow up appointments? If so, how did they go? Also, how is your rehab going? I hope all is well with you and I will continue praying for a good recovery.

April Southworth
Classified Sales Representative

———————

Hello,

It was great seeing you last week hope to see you again real soon. I think you look amazing for what you have been through. Please keep me updated and don't worry about work. We are rocking along and your teams are doing great. We all miss you.

Char

Shortly after my return home, I was honored with a visit from my Director, Charlotte Aaron, and fellow managers, Roxanne, Myrna, and Lana. Virtie was out sick that day, and Scott was holding the fort down at the office. As was the norm for the first few months, I would become overwhelmed with emotion upon seeing anyone for the first time since my rupture. The realization was that I might not have ever seen them again. "Live today like there is no tomorrow" suddenly cast a new light. No matter how many times I shared my story, I cried. Come to think of it, most have cried with me. These were healing times. Family and friends who loved me and cared for me surrounded me. They also hurt for me.

Word of mouth continued making rounds, and soon I would begin to hear from high school friends. Not particularly remarkable, as many of us have kept in close contact thirty-plus years after graduation. Billy called out of the clear blue sky one Sunday afternoon. He had heard the news of my rupture from one of his university students, who happened to be one of my coworkers. He arranged a visit one afternoon, and as soon as he walked in the front door, he held me tight, provided a "relief chest" to cry on. Just nine months earlier, the class of '77 had celebrated our thirtieth high school reunion. Billy and I sat at the dining room table, where I would share my story once again. No doubt, within minutes Billy would have me laughing. This was his gift, and I embraced it as though I had won the lottery. He would have made a perfect big brother. Liz, the closest of my high school confidants, along with a few other classmates, would visit shortly afterward. Again, each visit from family or friends lifted me up.

Jana, Karen, Luci, and Denise were regulars. Laughter would soon become more prominent than tears. There was always something going on at the office that would bring us amusement.

Five days after returning home, I would report to my primary care physician, Dr. Martin Wiesenthal, for a basic checkup and to have my dilantin levels measured and monitored. Joel and I made the trip back to the medical center and arrived early for the scheduled appointment. As usual, the waiting room was crowded, so we prepared ourselves for a long wait. As a general rule of thumb, we try very hard to not stare at people who have physical differences, and yet sometimes our curiosity gets the best of us. Approaching the counter to check in, I observed as people began turning around in my direction. The only reason this bothered me was because it apparently upset them. Oddly enough, my name was called within minutes after arriving, and Joel and I followed the nurse back to the exam room. We both took a seat as she slowly and cautiously asked, "What brings you in to see the doctor today?" It was one of those awkward moments when I thought I would burst out laughing! Instead, I explained this was a post-hospital follow-up appointment, after having suffered a ruptured brain aneurysm. She proceeded to tell me how wonderful I looked and began taking my vitals. Once she had documented my near-perfect blood pressure, pulse, and temperature, she informed me the doctor would be with us shortly and left the room, closing the door behind her. In the matter of a few minutes, I fought the urge to become weepy.

Dr. Wiesenthal knocked on the door, came in and introduced himself to Joel, and then turned his attention to me. He sat on his stool and rolled himself right in front of my chair. "How are you doing?" he asked, as we sat face to face. As hard as I tried to fight it off, my eyes began burning. "You look really good, Mickey. When I first saw you lying supine in that hospital bed…well, you gave everyone quite the scare," he continued. With Joel holding my hand and in between sobs, I managed to answer his questions. Yes, I was doing okay. Cried a lot, but doing okay. Yes, I was scheduled to follow up with Dr. Vardiman in a few days. No, I didn't have headaches or blurred vision. I was an emotional wreck, and he reassured me this was understandable, or perfectly normal, given the ordeal I lived through. "Perfectly normal" had not yet returned to my language.

After discussing a subsequent checkup for the following month, the nurse returned to chart various medications prescribed to me, along with the doses and frequency taken. To establish the dose of Dilantin that I needed to absorb, blood was drawn to determine where my natural Dilantin levels stood. One of the many purposes of this medication is the prevention of seizures following a head injury or surgery. The dose would increase from 200 milligrams daily to 500 milligrams daily before Doc was satisfied we were at a stable stage. In addition to other meds, this prescription read, "Take 100 mg in the morning, followed by 100 mg at lunch, and finally 300 mg at bedtime." To say I was alarmed at the number of pills I was taking every day would have been an understatement.

Dr. Wiesenthal was not an attending while I was in the hospital, as it took three days for the hospital to determine who my PCP was and then place the call to notify him. By then I was already under the watchful eye of several hospitalists at the Methodist. Dr. Wiesenthal did indeed make "social calls" to see how I was tracking and review my charts. Since I would be back under his charge upon release from the hospital, this was a well-executed plan on his part.

A few days later, we were back at the medical center once again to see Dr. Vardiman. Recalling the reaction of patients at my earlier appointment, I decided to wear a baseball cap. Joel parked, and we approached the very impressive TNI (Texas Neurosciences Institute) Building, where we would locate the offices of Neurosurgical Associates of San Antonio, P.A., where Dr. Vardiman practices with another half dozen brilliant neurosurgeons, including Dr. Donald L. Hilton.

Shortly after our arrival, Nurse Maria Byron, whom I had spoken to over the phone during an earlier Nimotop crisis, called me back. Her resolve was absolutely amazing, and she brought calm over me as soon as she introduced herself. Maria apologized as she explained Dr. Vardiman had been called away on an emergency.

It's funny how I could so easily relate. The purpose of this appointment was to remove all remaining staples on both my scalp and torso. She proceeded to gingerly extract the staples while observing and remarking that the incisions looked good. Following a bit of small talk, dos and don'ts, a few questions, and instructions for a CT scan to follow, we were on our way. My next appointment was scheduled for May, four weeks later.

Joel continued his work schedule, and Kyle was wrapping up his junior year in high school. This meant I would spend time alone, and my fears would become a manifestation from hell. Saturday nights proved to be the worst. The association of this rupture happening on a Saturday night had me spooked. Could it happen again? Would it happen again? When I became overly paranoid, all I had to do was pick up the phone. Frances would make the trip across town, no questions asked. So would Karen or Denise or Jana. Luci and Kim would visit and haul me off to dinner, where soup was the best I could do.

The day my BFF, Grace, arrived for a visit with a homemade chicken potpie in hand, I would slowly begin eating again. I've always been blessed with wonderful friends…most of whom have been in my life for years. When these friends surround you in your worst possible hour, you will see them in an entirely different light moving forward.

The second week of May, Dr. Vardiman signed a release for me to drive and also to return to work on a part-time basis effective June 2, 2008. This followed a routine check-up, where his nurse, Maria, would ask, "Have you had any seizures, Mickey?"

No, no seizures here. Oh my God! Was I going to have seizures? What is a seizure? Would I know if I was having a seizure?

Still taking anti-seizure medications, I was expected to be just fine. I arrived at this appointment with a list of questions. There were always questions. I began keeping a list so I wouldn't forget by the time my appointment rolled around. Questions provided answers, and answers provided reassurance. Answers, of course, also generated more questions.

## *Questions For*
## *Dr. Arnold Vardiman*

1. Please explain everything you did to me, including how my shunt and catheter work. I need to understand this.

2. What is the route of the drainage tube? Is there constant drainage?

3. What can you tell me about the "clicking" and "ringing" noise in my ears?

4. Why does the right side of my head/scalp get real numb? Why is it so sensitive? Should I be concerned that whatever position I lie in, my head starts to hurt?

5. Dilantin has been increased from 300 mg to 500 mg per day. Will I have to take this med long term?

6. My hearing has been super heightened; however, my vision is weaker than before. Is this temporary?

7. What is this indentation on the right-hand side of my head?

8. Do I have an aneurysm clip, or was it a clipped aneurysm?

9. In working on the right hand side of my brain, what function(s) does this regulate?

10. It's been over a month since I developed this pain in my side, with no diagnosis in sight. If it's not related to the shunt catheter (how did you determine), do you have any other suspicions?

11. Dr. Wiesenthal wants me to take Lyrica, but after reading up on this med, I'm apprehensive. Your thoughts?

12. Why did this happen to me?

Dr. Vardiman graciously answered every question and concluded this appointment with strict orders. I was ordered to walk. "I want you to walk forty-five minutes a day, six days a week. You don't have to walk fast, just walk," Doc advised me.

And so I did. But there was one tiny dilemma. I was afraid to venture out on my own, afraid something might happen and there wouldn't be anyone to help me if I fell, collapsed, or worse. But I wasn't afraid to walk around inside my home. And so I did. For forty-five minutes a day, I walked the inside perimeter of my house. Always the loyal companion, Toby followed me, each time stopping at the front door as we approached. It wasn't long before I had memorized the number of tiles that extended from one room to the next. I made a mental note of the baseboards that needed attention. I ran my finger alongside the barren walls. Then there were the games I concocted. Step on every other tile. Don't step on the cracks.

After the first week, Toby gave up on me. Up until this short-term disability leave, I was hardly ever home. Now I never *left* the house and walked around in circles all day long. Poor pup. The look in his eyes told me he knew something wasn't quite right in the land of Urias.

On his days off, Joel and I would venture outside for walks where I actually got some sunshine and fresh air. Toby was in tow.

Until I was given the green light to drive, Joel or Frances had been chauffeuring me to my various places of destination, i.e. doctors' appointments or the pharmacy. One afternoon I decided to wait outside, as Frances was en route to pick me up for yet another appointment. It was a bit chilly, so I unlocked my Kia to get inside, sit, and wait with the door slightly ajar. Within a few minutes, in my side-view mirror, I saw my neighbor Pat crossing the street. Although she and Chuck had been kept abreast of my progress through Joel, I had not seen these neighbors since *that* night. Pat had a look of concern on her face as she approached my truck and immediately asked if I was okay. She must have thought I was going to *attempt* to drive. I got out of the truck and explained to her I was waiting for my sister to pick me up. By now, Chuck was crossing the street and once again, my eyes started to water up. I recalled their presence that night and was ever so grateful to have them for neighbors. I hugged Pat, then Chuck. I thanked them for being there for Joel that night and for the years of friendship that we've shared as neighbors. They in turn reassured me that they would always be keeping an eye open for me and would be of any assistance if and whenever needed. Have you counted your blessings today? They returned home, and I got back into my car.

Shortly after being told I was able to drive again, it occurred to me that I hadn't been behind the wheel of my five-speed Sorento for about ten weeks. *It's all good*, I thought to myself. *Driving is like riding a bike, right? You never forget how, right?* Then I found myself questioning who in their right mind would allow someone to drive so soon after brain surgery.

My problem, as it turned out, was I didn't have a good understanding of how well I *was* doing. My pre-occupation with how *poorly* I *could* have been doing was all consuming.

One morning I decided to venture out and go have my nails done. It had been several weeks, and they were looking as bad as I had been feeling. The drive to the nail salon was a mere eight blocks from my house, and yes, it was like riding a bike. Aside from scaring the daylights out of everyone at the nail salon, all went well. Yes, I still looked pretty bad.

By mid May, I would make my first trip downtown to visit my workplace. After visiting with Greg and Laura, our security guards, I got on the elevator to head up to the fourth floor Classified Advertising Depart-ment. As soon as the elevator door opened, Denise made eye contact with me and approached me while I was experiencing an awkward moment. With an office the size of ours, I didn't know where to start and was very self-conscious of my appearance. She walked me to the conference room and laid down the law. "You don't need to be wandering all around this place…you stay here, and I'll e-mail everyone to let them know you're here, and they can come to you!" she preached.

In a matter of seconds, I was greeted with a del-uge of visitors as they stampeded toward the confer-ence room, lining up to greet me. As happy a moment as this was, yes, there were tears. Visitors from other departments made their way up to our office, and before I knew it, two hours had passed. I prepared to leave and promised to take another "field trip" the following week. These field trips would take place for the following three weeks, until I returned to work on June 2. My intent was to get out of the house, get some fresh air, and become reacquainted with my coworkers prior to going back to work, so there would be few disruptions when I did return to work.

Upon returning home from one of these visits, Charlotte called to tell me Tom Stephenson, our publisher, had heard I was in the building and wanted to see me next time I came by. Cabin fever had already gotten the best of me all the weeks I was convalescing at home, so all I needed was a reason to go and a full tank of gas. I called Tom's assistant and scheduled an appointment to see him.

A couple of days later, I was heading toward Tom's seventh-floor office and encountered Michael Marke, our director of finance. Michael seemed surprised to see me, and after brief pleasantries in the hallway, he asked, "Is it true you were calling your office from the intensive care unit?" Wow, I can't believe this fabricated story made its way from the Broadway building to the Avenue E building, as our departments were housed out of these two different locales. We said our good-byes, and I made my way to the publisher's office.

Upon cue from his executive assistant, I entered Tom's office with the trepidation of a schoolgirl walking into the principal's office. Quite honestly, I had never been in his office, although he poked his head into mine every now and again when he was in our building. Not quite sure how I should proceed, I approached Tom's desk as he got up and headed toward me. Should I shake his hand? Should I hug him like I do everyone else? He is, after all, the publisher for Pete's sake! We embraced and sat down in two facing chairs in front of his desk to visit. He inquisitively asked questions, and I answered them one by one. He confirmed that vicious rumor, the one that I had been calling the office while I was lying in ICU. Jokingly, I continued to vehemently deny this claim, although it was time to admit guilt. Most fascinating was his promise to allow me to take my trip to New York next year, since I wouldn't be able to as scheduled this year! It was a heartfelt encounter. I left his office feeling lifted and cared for. You are a good man, Mr. Tom Stephenson.

Prior to reporting back to work and as though going through a twelve-step program, I returned to the hospital. This time, however, as a visitor, not a patient. I wanted to visit the tenth-floor (NICU) nurses to thank them for taking care of me during those critical weeks. Frances had continued to tell me stories about how wonderful each and every one of them was. She spoke of one nurse in particular who nearly jumped over the nurse's station counter to get to my bedside when she saw me trying to sit up in my bed one afternoon. At that time, I was not supposed to be moving around, due to the magnetic contraption working with my drainage tube.

I felt compelled to see these men and women, to let them know I was okay, in part because of the impeccable care they provided. And maybe apologize to "Brian," who I called Brain after reading his hospital name badge incorrectly. *What a bizarre coincidence,* I thought. *What are the chances there would be a nurse named Brain taking care of a brain aneurysm patient such as myself?* Again…blame the drugs; I really *can* read.

I rode the elevator up to the tenth floor and walked to the double-electric doors that led to the NICU. I stood there, pondering the solitude, the sheer silence. The waiting room was empty, and I began to question if I was in the right place. After several minutes, I hit the automatic stainless steel plate that would open these double doors, where I would find myself in unfamiliar territory. How could I have spent as much time here as I had and not recall these surroundings? One of the nurses turned the corner and asked if she could be of assistance. It was her! It was the nurse who gave me that infamous bath in bed! I explained the purpose of my visit, and she escorted me to the nurse's station, all the while summoning the other nurses on duty. One by one, faces became recognizable. Again, I shared with them the reason I wanted to visit. I needed to thank them and was astonished that they were thanking me in return! "We never know what becomes of our patients once they leave us. We can only hope that they progress well, but for you to come back and allow us to see the fruits of our labor, thank you!" one of the nurses exclaimed. During this visit, they recalled the two different rooms I was housed in, raved about the doctors who cared for me, and rallied for my ongoing progress. And yes, they joked and laughed about the notorious phone calls I made to my office.

All support systems were beginning to take hold, but there was still something missing. I had a wealth of family and friends who would sit with me, cry with me, laugh with me…but they could not truly understand what I was going through. I trusted my doctors implicitly but was almost certain that none of them had personally had their brains bleed out, exposed during surgery, and pieced back together. I had to find someone who could *truly* relate.

My search for a brain aneurysm support group began, and the timing was nothing short of another miracle. I located the national Brain Aneurysm Foundation online (www.bafound.org), and was promptly directed to a newly founded local chapter in San Antonio. By newly founded, I mean to say that this small group had convened for their very *first* meeting in June 2008, which I missed by ten days of calling!

I met with Mayra, a survivor who founded the local San Antonio group, and arranged to attend the July meeting. We opted to meet one on one for lunch prior to the July gathering and ended up talking for four hours. She is also an aneurysm survivor, having discovered her aneurysm without rupturing. During our talk, she educated me on options for treating non-ruptured aneurysms. "They did what?" I asked in disbelief. Utilizing platinum coils to compact an aneurysm sounded absolutely amazing and very high tech, but I was shocked to discover how those coils get there! This would be my introduction to "Brain Aneurysms 101." Mayra gave me the low down on why and how she pursued founding the group and shared details of the first meeting, held days earlier. Wow, I thought. It's one thing to be involved in a group that shares similar interests or hobbies, but imagine how elite this group would be. Maybe this group would be able to help me rediscover that small piece of my inner-self that had gone missing. Surely, they would understand.

As amazing as the support group discovery turned out to be, even more so was a totally unexpected revelation from one of my coworkers. Upon my return to work, three months and one day following the rupture, there was a flurry of well wishers and "mother hens" hovering around my office, making certain I was okay. Released to work twenty hours per week for the first month, I was playing catch up and loving every minute of being back. Honestly, the preoccupation proved to be therapeutic.

Scott had taken on most of my responsibilities during my absence, and upon my return, he spent quality time getting me back up to speed with the products my teams and I were responsible for. He was also a regular at my office door, checking to see how I was doing, always asking if he could help in any way. On one visit, he came into my office and sat down to chat and asked me if I knew his mother had suffered a ruptured aneurysm! A bit shocked, I was ready to offer my apologies, when he continued. Her rupture had been seventeen years earlier, and she was alive and well. Up until this very moment, I was still relatively convinced my days were numbered. I had been so busy absorbing the mortality rates and possible permanent deficits that, like many people, I was prepared to make an awful, incorrect assumption. It took all of about fifteen seconds for this revelation to sink in, and my entire outlook was instantly changed. The weight of the world had been lifted off my shoulders. It reminded me that the simplest acts of kindness can change someone else's life. Thank you, Mr. Scott Butler. You played a major role in getting me on the path to redemption.

The July meeting for the newly formed support group in San Antonio was powerful. Although the group was small, I was introduced to five aneurysm survivors, and this would truly begin my quest to research and learn more about what I was dealing with. As much as I wanted to wish all of this away, truth be told, this was my life now. I had to learn to live with the fact that I was not the same person I was on February 29, 2008. What a leap year that turned out to be. There was no way for me to know that I would literally *leap* into a new me.

The group continued to grow, as our respective neurosurgeons distributed information about the survivors group to their aneurysm patients and families. We have become friends and confidants. We have been there for one another when undergoing procedures, including those to clip or coil aneurysms. As a group of "been there, done that," we were able to answer questions for family members sitting in the operating waiting room, frightened out of their minds. It has been a rewarding experience. To share our stories with these families…you can see the hope in their eyes. Seeing is indeed believing.

My first month at work was a blur. Time raced by. On a twenty-hours-per-week schedule, I was gaining strength, getting back in tune with my team, and making more progress with each passing day. I was even tempted to take a swing at the person who told me, "You're so lucky you only have to work twenty hours a week." But I didn't. She meant no harm and was totally oblivious to the insensitive remark that exited her mouth. I would have happily worked sixty hours a week again, in exchange for having my BA life back.

One morning, shortly after my arrival at the office, I felt a slight tickle inside my right ear. Perhaps, I thought to myself, I hadn't done a very good job drying it out after my morning shower. There was a medicine cabinet in the break room, which included cotton swabs. As I gingerly swabbed the inside of my ear, I withdrew the swab to discover blood on the cotton tip. Oh my gawd! I've sprung a leak! Silly as it sounds, I was truly mortified. When would this nightmare ever end?

An overactive imagination trumps a hypochondriac any day of the week. A visit to my faithful primary care physician was definitely in order. Dr. Wiesenthal verified a small collection of blood. Perplexed, and appearing a bit nervous himself, he in turn referred me to an ear, nose, and throat specialist, who upon further evaluation discovered a fresh laceration. It is not clear how I managed to scratch the inside of my ear hard enough to make it bleed. You would think one would remember doing so. Not true. Just very, very grateful it wasn't the leak that my imagination had manifested. Fear plays dirty.

A mere two weeks later, I would be walking to my office, probably too fast, when the rubber sole on my shoe caught the carpet and would send me flying. Gravity was working fine that day. I stopped falling right when I hit the floor! I can't remember ever seeing so many people move so fast. It only took a couple of seconds for me to realize I was okay, didn't hurt anywhere, and then I burst into laughter. I looked up at several puzzled faces while Karen was trying to lift me up by pulling me by my arm. It was a bizarre moment when I couldn't stop laughing; therefore her attempt to lift me from the floor was futile. I was as limp as a wet noodle. Once I was up and had reassured everyone I was fine, I went back to work, with only my pride bruised. Within a few days, I received a letter in the mail. Company policy states if you fall down while at work you needed to report to the company clinic for a drug-screening test. Now *that* was funny! I challenged the lab to rule out the drugs I *wasn't* taking. In the end, it was ruled that my fall was an accident. Case closed.

July turned into a glorious month, as I continued to gain momentum and had now been upgraded to work thirty hours per week. The morning of July 18, I sat down at the dining room table to finish my coffee and reflect on a birthday that might not have been. Once again, I began with the what-ifs. My dad remained in a fragile state, and I thought about how he would have suffered miserably through this day *if* I, his first-born child, had not survived.

As I began to apply makeup before going to work, tears welled up in my eyes. It's my birthday…I will not cry! Then I thought…what would Joel and the boys have done? While I was lost in thought, Kyle came over to the table to wish me a happy birthday. He kissed me on the cheek and presented me with a birthday card. They really do grow up too fast. I opened the card, and thought long and hard.

A beautiful sentiment, written by some faraway stranger, was conveying my son's wish for me. It's what I read in his handwriting that opened up the floodgates one more time…

> *I'll always be here for you Momma, to reassure you*
> *that everything will be okay.*
>
> *Love, Kyle*

August would bring an unexpected but thrilling invite. My dear friends Grace and Elvis would be traveling to the Chicago area to visit family. The wonder of this was that I too had family there! Grace's father, the incomparable Mr. Bill Hay, and my sister Toni actually live fifteen minutes from one another. So the invite would come to fruition. "Why don't you come with us?" Grace asked. Then Elvis chimed in and once again, I felt truly blessed. My initial reaction was "Yes, let's do it!" Only to be followed by, "Well…I don't know if I can." It had now been five months since my rupture, and although I felt well and stronger with each passing day, the thought of being thirty-five thousand feet in the sky suddenly terrified me. I wanted to do it, and I needed to do it. Make no mistake; I'm not afraid of flying. My dad was a career air force man, and for the first seven years of my life, we flew all over the world. I love flying; love the fact that I can be across the country in a matter of a couple of hours. My fear was that something might happen once we reached the highest of altitudes. Then what? I couldn't imagine dodging another bullet. Besides, you can only find a doctor on an airplane in the movies. Even if there was a bona fide doctor on board, what could he/she possibly do? Depending upon where we were, it would probably take forty-five minutes to conduct any kind of an emergency landing… stop it! I had become a victim of my own paranoia. A pre-fabricated fear, if you will. More importantly, I was getting on my own nerves. Yes, I was going to do this.

After getting the green light from Dr. Vardiman's office, with a reminder to avoid any magnetic devices, I was confident and ready to go. Besides, I would be traveling with friends who would move heaven and earth to watch over me. Tickets were purchased, bags were packed, and my medic alert bracelet was in place. Elvis and Grace arrived to pick me up in the wee hours of the morning for our 7:00 a.m. flight. After Elvis parked his truck and met us back in the terminal, we all headed toward security. Here's where it gets interesting. Due to my shunt implant, all magnetic devices are taboo and must be avoided at all costs. As Grace and Elvis headed to their screening area, I took a sharp right turn and approached the medical screening checkpoint. A very sweet and compassionate female TSA officer explained everything she was going to do, which in essence, was a complete body pat down. As she began to explain that she would start from the top of my head and work her way down, I felt compelled to tell her my head was not that of your average bear. She chuckled and asked, "What do you mean?" She probably thought I was implying that I wasn't all there. I didn't want her to feel this huge knot on the side of my head and think I had planted some explosive device. I warned her about the indentation on the other side of my head as well. She wasn't even slightly fazed. So the procedure began. I was not embarrassed, wasn't offended, and had only one request for undergoing this process when we returned home. May I request Tom Selleck next time? Please?

# AWARENESS – WHAT EVERYONE SHOULD KNOW

*"Let us not look back in anger or forward in fear,*
*but around us in awareness."*

James Thurber

The Brain Aneurysm Foundation was first established on August 19, 1994, and provides research funding for basic scientific research directed at early detection through the support of generous contributors.

Although my first visit to this website was indeed after the fact, it provided an enormous amount of information for me to review and become acclimated with. It really does help when you have the knowledge needed to comprehend the incomprehensible.

What Is A Brain Aneurysm?

A brain aneurysm is a weak bulging spot on the wall of a brain artery, very much like a thin balloon or weak spot on an inner tube.

## Brain Aneurysm Statistics

- An estimated 6 million people in the United States have an un-ruptured brain aneurysm, or 1 in 50 people.

- The annual rate of rupture is approximately 8 per 100,000 people or about 25,000 people.

- About 40 percent of all people who have a ruptured brain aneurysm will die as a result.

- Four out of seven people who recover from a ruptured brain aneurysm will have disabilities.

- Brain aneurysms are most prevalent in people ages 35 through 60, but can occur in children as well.

- Women, more than men, suffer from brain aneurysms at a ratio of 3:2.

- Ruptured brain aneurysms account for 3 to 5 percent of all new strokes.

## Warning Signs/Symptoms

Un-ruptured

- Cranial nerve palsy

- Dilated pupil

- Double vision

- Pain above and behind the eye

- Localized headache

- Drooping eyelid

Ruptured

- Localized or diffuse headache associated with one or more of the following:

- Nausea and vomiting

- Stiff neck

- Blurred or double vision

- Sensitivity to light (photophobia)

- Change in mental status or awareness

- Seizure

Risk Factors *that doctors and researchers believe contribute to the formation of brain aneurysms*:

- Smoking

- Hypertension

- Congenital, resulting from inborn abnormality in artery wall

- Drug use, particularly cocaine

- Infection

- Tumors

- Traumatic head injury

- Family history of brain aneurysms

- Other inherited disorders: Ehler's Syndrome, Polycystic Kidney Disease, and Marfan's Syndrome

- Presence of an arteriovenous malformation

Risk Factors *that doctors and researchers believe contribute to the* rupture *of brain aneurysms*:

- Smoking

- Hypertension

Courtesy Of:
The Brain Aneurysm Foundation
www.bafound.org
888-BRAIN02

In an effort to help raise awareness locally, the San Antonio Chapter of the Brain Aneurysm Foundation support group held the first Annual 5K Fun Run – 3K Walk for Brain Aneurysm Awareness and Hope. With the support of very generous sponsors and gung-ho volunteers, over $10,000 was raised and presented to the Brain Aneurysm Foundation. This event proved to be an eye opener in many ways. First, we had many more in attendance than expected, including several long-time aneurysm survivors who arrived at the event to show their support! For me, this validated the true meaning of survivor. Pulling together for one another because you can truly relate to and appreciate the long road that we will travel together.

On a more poignant note, an eighteen-year-old young woman traveled from out of state to attend the event in honor of her mother—lost to a brain aneurysm two years earlier. She had joined other family members who drove in from Laredo, and with matching T-shirts bearing her mother's photo, they all marched triumphantly to show their support.

Upon completion of the walk/run, it was a time for reflection. Those lost but not forgotten victims of brain aneurysms were remembered with the symbolic release of two hundred monarch butterflies. It was truly a sight to behold, and one could not help but to become misty-eyed. As grateful as we are for those who beat the odds and survived, we can never forget those less fortunate, including the families they left behind.

This is why it is imperative that everyone understands the odds, the risks, and what to do if you suspect you or your loved one is experiencing any of the symptoms of an aneurysm. Time is indeed relevant.

Understanding History, Early Detection, and Screening Methods:

It Could Save Your Life!

## Family History

- Familial intracranial aneurysms are generally defined as the presence of two or more family members among first and second-degree relatives with proven aneurysmal SAH (subarachnoid hemorrhage) or incidental aneurysms.

- The incidence of familial aneurysms among SAH patients is 6 to 20 percent.

- Familial intracranial aneurysm is defined as two or more blood relatives who possess intracranial aneurysms.

- The familial occurrence suggests a genetic component and the possibility of a genetically determined defect of the arterial wall.

- Several studies suggest that individuals with familial intracranial aneurysms are more likely to have multiple aneurysms and that these aneurysms are more likely to rupture at a smaller size than those patients with an isolated aneurysm.

- Treatment considerations are different for patients with familial aneurysms than for patients with an unruptured isolated aneurysm.

- The Familial Intracranial Aneurysm Study (FIA) has recruited a number of families and their goal is to identify genes that underlie the development and rupture of intracranial aneurysms.

- The National Institute of Neurological Diseases funded the largest genetic linkage study to date. The study includes twenty-six clinical centers that have broad experience in clinical management and imaging patients with intracranial aneurysms. The study will recruit 475 families with affected sib pairs or with multiple affected relatives through retrospective and prospective screening of potential subjects with an intracranial aneurysm.

- An important aspect of the genetic study is the study of environmental factors in disease risk such as smoking. Nearly 80 percent of patients with an Intracranial Aneurysm (IA) have a history of smoking at some time in their life. Not all individuals who smoke develop IA. Smoking may increase the risk of IA for individuals with specific genotypes at IA susceptibility.

## Early Detection and Screening

Brain aneurysms can be similar to heart attacks. Just like a person may have no warning of an impending heart attack, there almost is never a warning that a brain aneurysm is about to rupture. Fortunately, through imaging screening techniques, individuals at high risk of harboring a brain aneurysm can be identified easily with non-invasive imaging tests.

Risk factors for developing brain aneurysms include cigarette use; disorders of the body's structural proteins (Ehlers-Danlos syndrome, Marfan syndrome); fibromuscular dysplasia; chronic hypertension; history of cerebral aneurysms in closely related family members; use of cocaine, crack, or amphetamines; and polycystic kidney disease. Our recommendation is for any individual over the age of twenty-five who has a first-degree blood relative (e.g., mother, father, brother, sister) with a brain aneurysm be screened for aneurysms.

Two quick and safe ways to screen for aneurysms include MRI with MRA (magnetic resonance imaging with angiography) and CT with CTA (computed tomography with angiography). Images that are obtained during these studies will reliably detect aneurysms as small as 2 mm. There are advantages and disadvantages of each of these types of studies.

MRA images are generated as a result of disturbances in a strong magnetic field. Excellent pictures of the brain itself are obtained and reasonably good pictures of the major arteries are as well. This is a good way to do an initial "screen." These are very safe tests as no radiation is used, but the quality and detail of the images are not as good as CTA or catheter angiography. In addition, it might take as long as forty minutes for a patient to complete one of these studies, and patients who are claustrophobic frequently need to be sedated, as the confines of the machine induce a sense of claustrophobia.

CTA images are created by injecting an iodine-based dye into the vein of the arm. As it passes from the vein to the heart and then pumps to the brain, X-rays are passed through the head, and images are created. This is a very fast test that takes only a few minutes to perform, and the quality and detail of the images are excellent. The downside is that it does expose the patient to X-ray radiation and iodine, which in some patients can lead to an allergic reaction. Usually, CTA is reserved as a follow-up study to an MRA study if an aneurysm is detected and there is a need to collect more information on the aneurysm. This additional information allows for a more detailed conversation with the physician on the need for treatment and what types of treatment options are available.

Catheter-based angiography is not a good initial test for screening, as the small risk of this procedure does not justify its use when MRA and CTA are effective in this role.

Information courtesy of
The Brain Aneurysm Foundation
www.bafound.org
888-BRAIN02

Awareness can and will save lives. Not only does it equate to more knowledge, but it also makes you super keen about a subject matter you may have not paid attention to before. Before my personal rupture, I had only heard of two other cases. Since my rupture and because of the awareness brought on by said rupture, it seems like I hear about brain aneurysms at least twice a week. Whether it is on the news, a reference made on a sitcom, or by someone I work with, I have learned more about this debilitating condition in the past year than I ever imagined possible. Knowledge is indeed power, and even though it is after the fact in my case, I pray that others are well informed. If need be, seek medical attention that can not only spare your life but may also allow a treatment that is minimally invasive. Nobody wants his or her head taken apart, however if it turns out to be a matter of life or death, chances are very good that you will sign the consent forms.

# My Perfect Rainbow

*"My life is my message."*
Mahatma Ghandi

October brought a change of seasons and more promising news. My follow-up appointment with Dr. Vardiman was truly remarkable. He was quite pleased with both the CT scan results and my overall progress. Upon review of my medications, I had now been removed from all but one anti-seizure medication, Dilantin. Doc would refer me to a neurologist who, in turn, would conduct a prolonged EEG (electroencephalography) assessment. I had never suffered a seizure. Not before, during, or after my aneurysm rupture. Was I truly prone to suffering seizures after this ordeal and subsequent surgery now? We would soon find out.

On December 12, I reported to the clinic of Dr. John Luther, where his assistant would proceed to glue a total of twenty-one electrodes to various points of my scalp. For the next forty-eight hours, I would wear this contraption, as it monitored brain activity while both awake and asleep. As I left the clinic, I pulled my hood up and over my wire-encrusted head and gave thanks it had now become dark outside. With two-inch spiked new growth hair and a mass of wires adhered to my noggin, I was reminiscent of a techno version of Medusa. Joel and Kyle were even more amused upon my return to the house; Toby, however, was just plain spooked.

Just when I had finally gotten my sleep groove back, this getup would jolt it. Again, wires all over the place connected to a recording device that I wore everywhere, including bed. Try rolling over a brick in bed; this is what I was contending with. Oh well, it would only be for two nights and any naps I might take.

Bright and early the following morning, I scared the bejesus out of my brand new, hadn't-even-met-her-yet next-door neighbor when I ventured outside to get my paper, in full regalia. I tried to reassure her everything was okay and told her we should get together for coffee sometime. Who can blame her? To this day, whenever we run in to each other, she is bolting faster than lightning.

The jokes and minor inconvenience were well worth the spectacular news that arrived just in time for Christmas. Here, in a nutshell, were Dr. Luther's findings.

> This prolonged digital EEG monitoring did not capture any typical clinical spells or seizures of clinical concern.

Dr. Luther would now begin a six-week process of having me weaned from this last medication.

Merry Christmas to me!

The holidays took on a whole new meaning, as I now had a childlike appreciation for everything. With each passing day and each passing milestone, I continued to gain strength and, more importantly, conviction. Well, I always had conviction, but it was taken from me on that fateful night. As the months continued to roll by, my fear of suffering another rupture began to wane. Yes, more progress was made each day, and each of my doctors had nothing but good reports to give me. How had I become my own worst enemy? The time had finally arrived, as I began to believe in myself again—the first step to believing anyone else.

March 1, 2009, was my one-year "Annie-versary" and truly a joyous occasion to celebrate. Most of the support group reconvened at Pickrell Park, the site of our earlier awareness event, to celebrate. By now, there was much more laughter, and the only tears were those of happiness or emphatic laughter. We still talk about the when, where, how, and why...but we have learned more about acceptance and continue to work on coming to terms with our aneurysms, ruptures, ongoing healing processes, and so on. As I sat on the park bench, I couldn't help but compare this beautiful day with *that* day, exactly one year ago. What if? What if I had known beforehand that I was an aneurysm carrier? What if everyone had the opportunity to find out before a rupture? What can I do moving forward? Is this my purpose?

For the longest time, I didn't want to talk about my condition. If I talked about it, it meant I had to relive it. I am so over that now. It is what it is, and I can't change the past. I can only live for today and hope for tomorrow.

The statistics remain all too sobering. Not long after my return to work, I stood outside my office door and pondered the numbers. One in fifty people have an aneurysm. There were fifty-four team members in my department. Coincidence? What are the odds? These *are* the odds. Unfortunately, I fit the profile, as I displayed many of the characteristics of an aneurysm carrier. Upon my recovery, I had some very serious decisions to make if I wanted to heal properly and completely. Yes, I modified my diet. I quit smoking. I started a long overdue exercise program. Everything my doctor had been pleading with me to do for years. What a concept.

Like many, I truly believed myself to be bulletproof. Nothing bad would ever happen to me, as I was reasonably healthy. We cannot determine whether or not this aneurysm was genetically inherent or brought on by high blood pressure, stress levels, weight, smoking, childhood injuries, etc. I won't risk the chance of developing another. Let's do a better job of taking care of ourselves. And while we're at it, let's help take care of each other.

After all, how often do we have the opportunity to witness *a perfect rainbow?*

*Expressions that crack me up...*

"Not tonight dear; I have a craniotomy-ache."

"I need that cookie like I need a hole in my head!"

"It doesn't take a brain surgeon to figure that out!"

"May I pick your brain for a second?" (Duh...no.)

"I really have had brain surgery. What's your excuse?"

*A few Survivors you may recognize...*

Joe Biden—Vice President
of the United States of America

Mario Batali—Chef (The Food Network)

Quincy Jones—Musician/Producer

Sharon Stone—Actress

*In Closing...*

Life isn't about waiting for the storm to pass;
It's about learning how to dance in the rain.

and

Live simply. Love generously. Care deeply.
Speak kindly. Leave the rest to God.

Authors Unknown